DIET AND WORKOUT PLANNER

HOW TO STAY HEALTHY AND GET FIT FOR LIFE

Dr. Robertino Bedenian

Diet and Workout Planner: How to Stay Healthy and Get Fit for Life

Dr. Robertino Bedenian

Published by Dr. Robertino Bedenian, 2024.

While every precaution has been taken in the preparation of this book, the publisher assumes no responsibility for errors or omissions, or for damages resulting from the use of the information contained herein.

DIET AND WORKOUT PLANNER: HOW TO STAY HEALTHY AND GET FIT FOR LIFE

First edition. January 27, 2024.

ISBN: 979-8224728671

Written by Dr. Robertino Bedenian.

Also by Dr. Robertino Bedenian

Fitness Over 60 For Women – How to Stay Fit And Healthy As You Age

Does Back Pain Go Away? 10 Answers To The Most Acute Back Pain Issues

Massage Bible - A Beginners Guide To Western And Eastern Massage Therapy

Going Vegan - How To Vegan Without Going Crazy

Chiropraktik - Was Steckt Eigentlich Dahinter?

Massagen: Ein Überblick Über Westliche Und Östliche Massagetechniken

Natuerlich Abnehmen, Schlank Und Endlich Fit Sein

P.S. Ich Liebe Dich: Wenn Liebe So Einfach Wäre

Was Tun Bei Rückenschmerzen, Bandscheibenvorfall Und Ischiasschmerzen: 10 Antworten Zu Den Häufigsten Fragen Bei Rückenschmerzen

Was Tun Gegen Schlafapnoe, Schlafstörungen Und Schnarchen

Self-Help Books for Women – How to Overcome Depression, Anxiety, Divorce, Addiction, and Trauma

Your Super Gut Feeling Restored – How to Restore Your Life Energy and Overall Health from The Inside Out

Diabetes How to Help: Everything You Need to Know About Diabetes Type 1 and Type 2

Diet and Workout Planner: How to Stay Healthy and Get Fit for Life

Everything I Know About Love

The Sleep Easy Solution Book: How to Stop Sleep Apnea, Snoring, and Sleep Disorders

Watch for more at https://booksummarypublishing.com.

Table of Contents

Download Your FREE Gift Now

How to Decide on The Right Weight Loss Plan!

As a way of saying "thank you" for your purchase, I'm going to share with you a

FREE Gift that is exclusive to readers of "Diet and Workout Planner".

It will help you turn your life around even faster with a diet and exercise regimen that works!

<u>Go Here to Check it Out:</u>

https://goingveganhealthbenefits.com/ weight-loss-plan

Obesity Rates Continue to Trend Up in U.S.

Percentage of U.S. adults who are obese based on height and weight survey

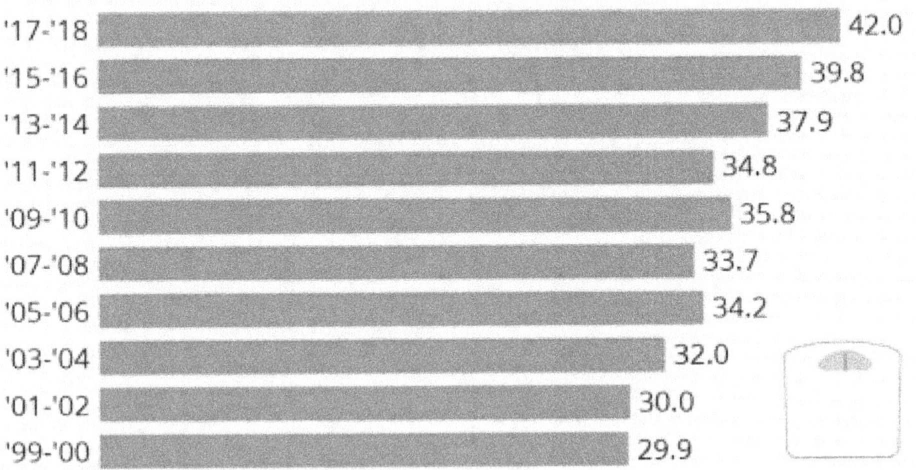

Data collected by CDC based on survey of 5,000 U.S. adults

Source: Centers for Disease Control and Prevention

 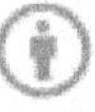 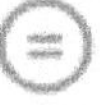

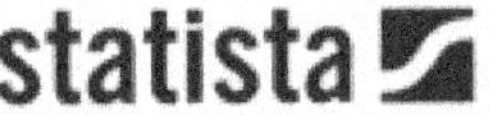

Chapter 1: Introduction

As a fitness trainer, my students often come up with the question of how to lose weight successfully and effectively. Admittedly, this question is asked far more often by women. Although men are still much more often overweight than women, the desire for an ideal weight seems to be more anchored in women. The dream of the perfect body occupies people all over the world. It is an *international* issue, so to speak. Being overweight is not only an aesthetic problem but is also associated with a variety of health problems. Most people who want to lose weight agonize over the best weight loss program they should undergo to achieve their goals. Many are already overwhelmed by the offers. They seem to have no plan and/or no strategy and are therefore often susceptible to the so-called miracle cures and miracle pills. This book, however, wants to be very plain about that issue: When you have finished reading this book, you will know EXACTLY how you can best lose weight, what you should avoid in order not to gain weight, and how you can also become and remain physically fit. You can achieve your goal of losing weight in different ways. Therefore, this book wants to show you different ways. However, it will also point out the methods that you should avoid at all costs. In this context, it will also address some of the traps you might fall into in your quest for the perfect weight loss plan, such as diet pills, eating disorders, and the typical nutrition myths. With this in mind, the health consequences of these traps are also addressed. To help readers of this book avoid these mistakes right from the start, let's begin our search for the perfect weight loss plan by identifying which methods do NOT work!

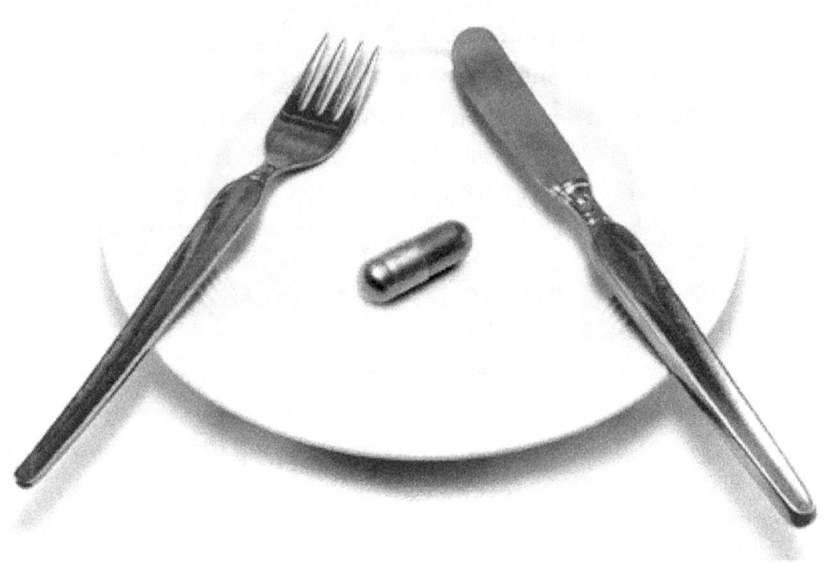

Chapter 2: Diet Programs You Should Absolutely Avoid!

2.1 The truth about diet pills

As far as access to diet pills is concerned, people of the 21st century have it far easier than previous generations. Back in the 50s, 60s, and 70s, diet pills were usually derivatives of amphetamines. They are also popularly known as "speed." These pills addicted millions of people and destroyed hundreds of thousands of lives. What made them particularly dangerous was their effect because on the one hand they actually worked, making many succumb to the temptation to use them, time and again, to quickly lose a few pounds. On the other hand, they came at a high price: First, they were indeed expensive, and second, they were as addictive as a classic drug. Nowadays, diet pills often don't even promise weight loss. Their addictive potential has diminished, but so has their effect. Losing weight this way is more than unlikely. Of course, nowadays you will still find some diet pills that help reduce weight. However, it should be noted that most of them have very alarming side effects so that the risk-benefit ratio is anything but balanced. Diet pills that are advertised in commercials, in a magazine, or on a billboard, for example, are usually a complete farce. They hardly deliver what they promise. But even if this were the case, you would pay far too high in terms of side effects.

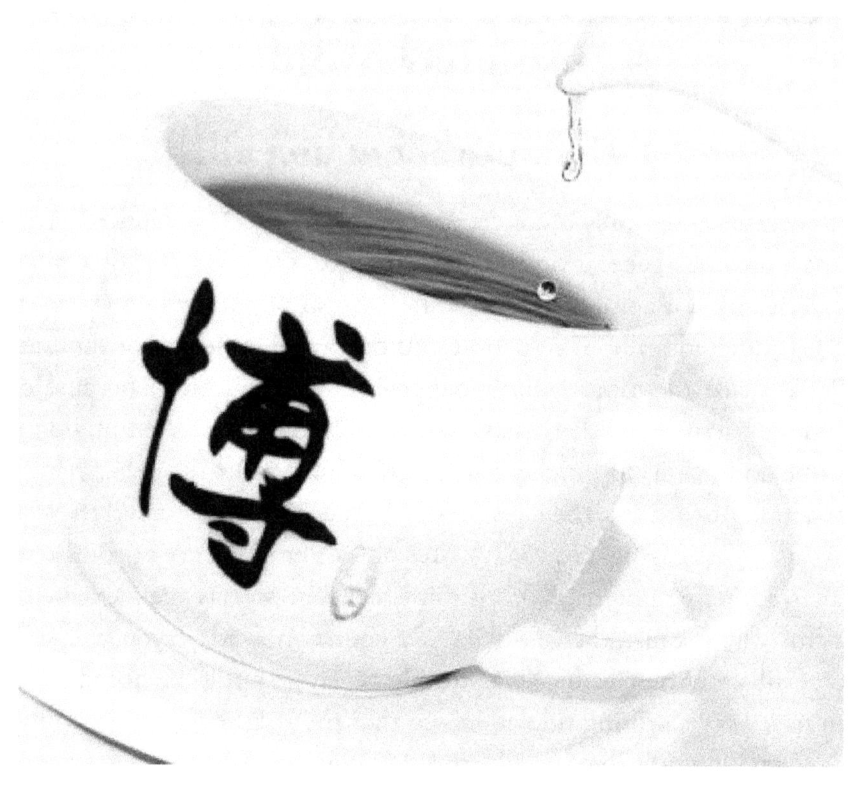

2.2 Hands off laxatives (laxatives)

A popular weight loss supplement is also available on the market in the form of tea. You will find almost in any grocery store the so-called "slimming tea". At first glance, it certainly does not seem to miss its effect. But appearances are deceiving because one of its effects is frequent bowel movements, i.e. slimming teas have a laxative effect. This gives sufferers the feeling of a body cleansing taking place. That's why they believe that they are purifying their bodies and thus getting rid of the toxins in their bodies. However, this is only half the truth: Slimming tea also contains herbs that are natural laxatives. These include *aloe, senna, rhubarb, cascara, sea buckthorn,* and *castor oil.* These are products derived from plants and have been used since ancient times for their effectiveness in treating constipation and stimulating bowel movements.

Cascara, castor oil, and senna are substances known as non-prescription laxatives and are also considered medicines. Scientific studies show that laxative-induced diarrhea excretes excess calories only to an insignificant extent. The effect is therefore quite negligible for the following reason: Laxatives do not affect the small intestine, where most calories are absorbed. Instead, they affect the large intestine. When laxatives are taken in large amounts and over a long period, they can lower the body's fat absorption. In most cases, this leads to severe diarrhea. Abuse of laxatives is common practice among people suffering from bulimia and anorexia. This will be discussed further in the next section. You may very probably lose some weight by the regular use of laxatives, but they also cause permanent damage to the gastrointestinal tract while weakening and softening the bones. This condition is called *osteomalacia* (softening of the bones). Drinkers of slimming teas often advocate taking them in part because slimming teas are often cheaper and taste better than other laxatives that are freely available on the market. Other people who suffer from eating disorders such as bulimia and anorexia prefer slimming teas because they work quickly and promote a liquid bowel movement. Women seem to be particularly susceptible to the effects of slimming teas. Although it has not yet been proven that slimming teas affect the menstrual cycle and fertility, care should be taken to prevent weight loss from occurring too quickly. Pregnant women are advised against taking laxatives of any kind. Herbalists also advise pregnant women and those who want to become pregnant against the use of senna and other herbal products with laxative effects. One should generally be cautious about the product descriptions of slimming teas, as the brand-name labeling of slimming teas on the market can often be misleading. For example, you can always find product descriptions that deliberately avoid the term "laxative" or "laxative" and instead often label their laxative effects as "natural colon cleansing," which of course sounds much better and less worrisome. Some even have the phrase "low calorie" on their label. In fact, these products contain no calories or nutrients unless they have been sweetened.

In addition to their laxative effect, other much more worrisome side effects occur from taking slimming teas when they are taken over a long period. These include nausea, stomach cramps, vomiting, diarrhea, fainting, rectal bleeding, electrolyte imbalances, and dehydration. The latter can even be fatal. Some testimonials also show that excess use of stimulant laxatives can cause severe constipation, which can even last for several years. The reason for this is that the bowel can no longer perform its function resulting sometimes in the entire removal of intestines.

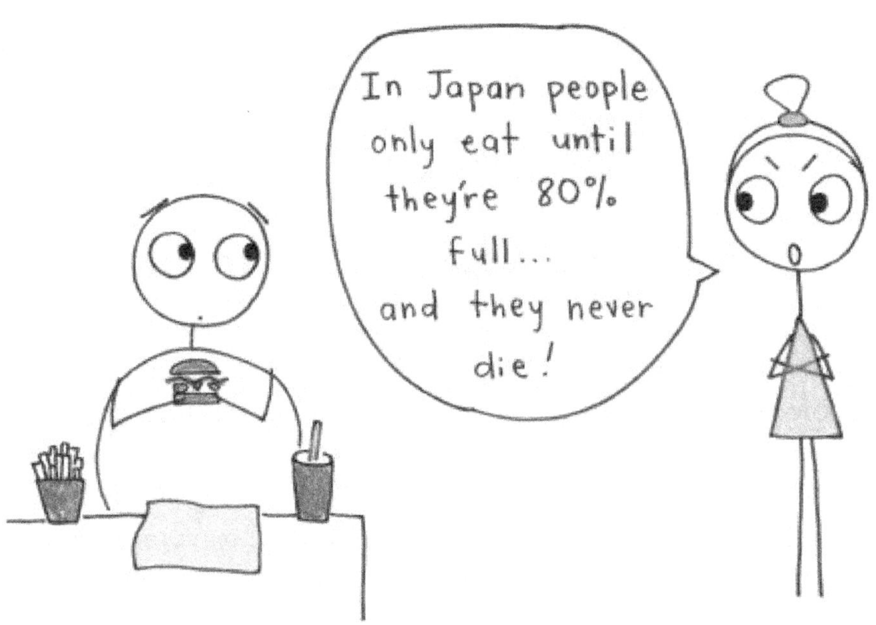

In Japan people only eat until they're 80% full...
and they never die!

Chapter 3: Dangerous Eating Disorders

A lot of people look down on people who have eating disorders like *bulimia*, *pica*, or *anorexia*. However, what many don't know is that these disorders are serious *mental* illnesses that are difficult to cure. In fact, testimonials show that more than 80% of people who suffer from bulimia never get better.

3.1 Body Dysmorphic Disorder

In order to understand the two most common eating disorders, it is first necessary to recognize the underlying condition that causes them: Body Dysmorphic Disorder. However, not everyone who suffers from body dysmorphic disorder necessarily develops bulimia, anorexia, or pica. Body dysmorphic disorder is characterized by the inability of sufferers to see themselves as they are. When these people look at themselves in the mirror, they don't see themselves, but something they can't stand. A typical example would be a spindly woman or man who looks in the mirror and sees an overweight person.

You might think that this is crazy, but these people actually see a physically different person in the mirror. In this perceptual disorder lies the real cause of most eating disorders, which lead these people to use not only ineffective but above all dangerous methods to lose or gain weight, because these people are not satisfied with the body they perceive.

3.2 Bulimia (Bulimia Nervosa)

Bulimia, also called binge eating disorder, is an eating disorder that arises from the desire to be thin.

The typical characteristics of bulimia sufferers are the so-called ravenous *hunger pangs*, against which countermeasures, such as self-induced vomiting, are immediately taken to avoid weight gain. Individuals with this disorder may or may not suffer from body dysmorphic disorder.

It is characteristic of bulimia sufferers that they often succumb to a kind of "eating frenzy" which, however, then leads them to feel guilty and therefore subsequently induce their vomiting.

Common symptoms of this disease include rotten teeth from contact with acid vomit, a poorly developed gag reflex (pharyngeal reflex), scarred or scraped knuckles that rub against the teeth, peculiar eating habits, and constantly going to the bathroom after every meal. In addition, they are also conspicuous for a strange pattern of behavior, such as taking a bite and then spitting it out. Of particular concern is that their fluid intake drops sharply, leading to a marked deterioration in overall health. Unfortunately, as mentioned earlier, most people with this disease do not fully recover. It is a *mental* illness and as such, its treatment success is dependent on the support of family members and competent psychiatric counseling. If you know someone who suffers from bulimia, or if you feel that you are a victim of this illness, you should immediately contact a knowledgeable counselor and talk to your family about it.

Through bulimia, losing weight ultimately remains a utopia. Rather, the pathological eating behavior puts the body into a kind of "emergency mode" and all calories taken in during cravings are immediately stored as fat.

3.3 Anorexia Nervosa (Anorexia)

As for the so-called *anorexia,* this disease is due to the desire to become thinner. This disease is somewhat less complex than bulimia but is much more likely to have a fatal outcome. Anorexic people simply tend not to eat. They often exercise intensely and eat only tiny meals, if any. A typical trend among anorexics is to dip cotton balls in yogurt and eat them, thus suppressing their hunger pangs. Anorexia is one of the mental illnesses with the highest fatality rate. Unlike bulimia, almost all people with this disease also suffer from body dysmorphic disorder. In other words, they are unable to assess their physical condition. Their perceptual disorder causes them to ALWAYS think of themselves as overweight.

Symptoms of anorexia include the following: Extreme weight loss, severely underweight, listlessness, lack of concentration, fainting spells, downy hair, severe constipation, dehydration, darkening of the skin around the eyes, and eventually death. Anorexics eventually die of starvation. They exhibit the exact same symptoms as those of starving people. They suffer from a complete lack of nutrients and electrolytes, which are vital for maintaining bodily functions. If the condition is not treated, anorexics can succumb to a heart attack or stroke.

In this case, I would like to point out that in case you know someone who may be suffering from this disease, or you yourself are in danger of falling victim to it, seek medical advice immediately. Anorexics who are not treated in a timely manner have a higher-than-average mortality rate. In almost all cases, this disease is based on a body dysmorphic disorder that is extremely difficult to treat.

3.4 pica

Although *pica* is undoubtedly a serious disease, it is generally considered to be one of the more harmless eating disorders. It can be caused by any number of psychological factors. Unfortunately, pregnant women suffer from pica for some unknown reason sometimes. Pica sufferers tend to eat things that are generally considered inedible or even disgusting.

Usually, these eating habits are rather harmless, but in extreme cases can lead to death. Those who suffer from pica develop a craving for things that are not food in any way. Some eat dirt, others paint or small stones as well as everyday objects. This disease can even manifest itself in such a way that some people start eating metal coins resulting in an entire intoxication of the body.

Pica is a very serious disease because it is impossible to predict what the sufferer will ingest. This mental disorder is not comprehensible with common sense. Consuming dangerous things like antifreeze or bullets is due to a very serious mental disorder. In this case, medical help should be sought immediately if you happened to know people in your environment who exhibit these behavioral abnormalities.

Chapter 4: Nutrition Myths You Should Know About

4.1 Drinking Diet Drinks Makes You Lose weight

The myth that diet drinks make you lose weight is still quite well spread today, as diet drinks initially certainly deliver what they promise: Diet sodas have no calories, and that's why they certainly make you lose weight. However, the downside is that they are rich in sodium, dyes, preservatives and other chemicals. Let's talk about sodium for a moment: Sodium is essential for the body to survive. However, only a certain daily amount is necessary for it. In the United States, as well as in many other countries, diet is very high in sodium: Sauces, fried foods, frozen foods, and every type of canned food are filled to the brim with sodium. Against this background, sodium consumption far exceeds daily requirements. Therefore, regular intake of diet drinks eventually leads to the body being loaded with an "overdose" of sodium. Because diet drinks are virtually calorie-free, many often tend to consume twice as many diet drinks as "regular" drinks. Excess sodium causes the body to absorb too much water. On the one hand, taking diet drinks prevents them from consuming sugar, which is abundant in "normal" drinks. On the other hand, however, they will cause sufferers to have an excessive amount of water in their bodies and stimulate appetite, as diet drinks appeal to the taste buds. This, in turn, will cause sufferers to eat even more than would be the case if they were drinking only the classic drinks or even plain water. Flavored water is a much better solution. Although this also stimulates the appetite, it is healthier.

4.2 Eating in The Evening Makes You Fat

To put this straight right at the beginning: In fact, this is not true! It has not been proven that eating before bedtime has a different effect on nutrient and fat absorption than eating at other times. This is because assuming that insulin release after carbohydrate intake particularly favors fat storage at night has not been proven. However, if you have already eaten plenty of calories during the day, you should prepare something light in the evening to keep your "energy balance" in check. Some people can start their day with a cup of coffee, eat a small snack at noon, and then have a warm meal in the evening. It is crucial to listen to your biorhythm. As for me, I follow the rule: "Eat like a king in the morning, like a citizen at noon, and like a beggar in the evening." However, this maxim is not universal. It comes from times when people worked hard, especially physically. Those who had to work hard in the morning should also treat themselves to a sumptuous breakfast. Those who eat the main meal of the day in the evening do not necessarily become fat. It depends on the total amount of energy you consume.

4.3 Carbohydrates Are The Real Thickeners

One of the most widespread myths is that carbohydrates are the real thickeners. The danger of this thesis is that it tempts many people to give up carbohydrates as much as possible. People who did this exhibited several very serious disease symptoms over time, even including kidney failure. Carbohydrate-rich foods were replaced as much as possible with protein-rich foods. However, carbohydrates provide the energy for physical and mental activities. Because protein is not the only vital nutrient that your body cannot do without. A lack of nutrients and protein-containing products will seriously affect the body's functions sooner or later. You should, therefore, take the claims made by proponents of a low-carbohydrate diet for weight loss with great misgivings. Your body will always use carbohydrates as its *primary* source of energy. Using protein as an energy source, on the other hand, is a last-ditch attempt to gain energy to still somewhat maintain bodily functions. Accessing your body's fat stores is something your body will generally reserve for "emergencies" when both carbohydrates and protein are depleted or no longer available in sufficient quantities. So, the problem is not the carbohydrates you consume. Rather, what matters is how many you consume, how you consume them, and how they are distributed throughout your body.

Carbohydrates are found almost everywhere. However, not all carbohydrates are the same! A distinction is made between *complex* and *simple* carbohydrates. *Complex* carbohydrates are found in vegetables, fruits, potatoes, legumes (peas, beans, lentils, etc.), whole grain bread, whole grain cereals, whole grain rice, whole grain pasta, and millet. These carbohydrates provide plenty of energy, provide the body with nutrient-rich calories and fiber, keep you full for a long time, and are slow to enter the bloodstream. These carbohydrates are consumed slowly in the body, namely as needed. For this reason, they are completely burned by the body over time and are not converted into fat. With this in mind, you could say that these carbohydrates burn slowly, like "carb briquettes".

Simple carbohydrates are found in sugar, honey, sweet fruits, sweets, pastries, cakes, light bread, toast, cola, soda, fruit juice, etc. They can quickly provide short-term energy to the body, but only provide it with many empty and nutrient-poor calories, only keep you full for a short time and quickly enter the blood. These carbohydrates burn quickly like newsprint compared to complex carbohydrates. Such carbohydrates, and especially those found in refined sugars, on the other hand, are completely converted into fat by the body almost immediately. This is because your body doesn't usually consume a large amount of sugar at one time, and, instead of evenly distributing the excess sugar throughout the body, the excess sugar is stored in fat stores for future "emergencies." As you can see, carbohydrates are not the true thickeners per se. However, if you overconsume the "wrong" carbohydrates, they will contribute to gaining weight. Therefore, make sure that your diet consists primarily of complex carbohydrates. Instead of cakes, ice cream, sweets, soda pop, and white bread, eat beans, brown rice, whole-grain bread, vegetables, and (non-sweet) fruits.

THE FOOD PYRAMID

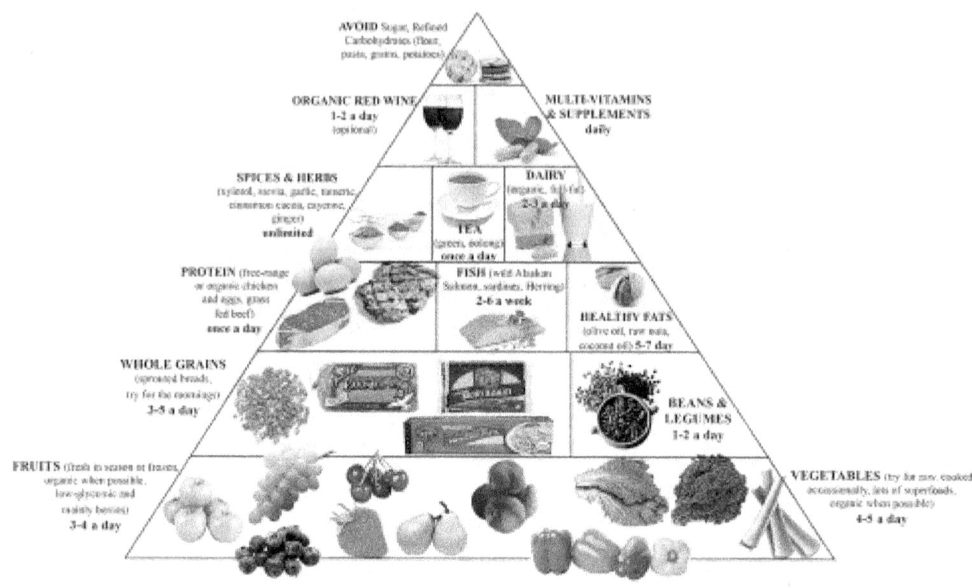

Chapter 5: Diet Change As New Lifestyle

First of all, I would like you to notice that the title of this chapter was not chosen by chance. If you seriously desire to lose weight and maintain your desired weight, then you must indeed also be prepared to change your diet. The word "diet" often suggests to most people I have talked to the character of a temporary change in eating habits to achieve the desired goal of weight loss. However, this is not the case. Rather, it is a final decision to completely change one's diet. With this in mind, it may indeed be a new *lifestyle* that you should be willing to pursue. Please do not underestimate this attitude! Because otherwise, you are in danger of losing your desired weight again very quickly after having achieved it so painstakingly. A temporary change in diet will only lead to temporary results. What you surely want, however, is a weight at which you feel permanently comfortable. There are a lot of resources available on the internet for you to decide which diet plan suits you best. However, as you are reading this book right now suggests being a result of that research. However, the most important thing is that you implement this diet plan *permanently*. Otherwise, you will be stuck with the so-called "yo-yo effect". Then let's get right to work on how you can best start your diet change!

5.1 What You Should Do Without!

You probably won't enjoy this chapter too much if the following things are already part of your diet. In this case, please keep your goal in mind. It will be worth it in the end! There are things that you should completely banish from your diet plan. These include the following things:

a) Trans fats - The Silent Killers

Trans fats are created by producing fats from liquid vegetable oil. Heating these fats produces artificial trans fatty acids and thus harmful fat. The particular advantage is that they become spreadable this way and can thus be used in a variety of ways. Fats made this way also have a much longer shelf life, making them very popular in restaurants and snack bars. Have you ever wondered why French fries always look so appetizingly brown in restaurants and snack bars?

This is due to the trans fats that the owners use. Regrettably, trans fats are almost everywhere in modern food. Aside from the aforementioned French fries, they are often found in chips, fried foods like chicken wings, in doughnuts and puff pastry, instant soups, gravy sauces, sausage, and even in granola bars or breakfast cereals. Regardless of whether you want to lose weight, you should avoid trans fats at all costs. Numerous studies have shown that they are responsible not only for obesity but also for other diseases, such as catastrophic metabolic disorders, a significant increase in "bad" cholesterol (LDL) with a simultaneous decrease in "good" cholesterol (HDL), noticeable susceptibility to inflammation in the body, increase in vascular diseases that significantly increase the risk of stroke or heart attack. The odds are that developing diabetes is also favored by the consumption of trans fats. Trans fats are often referred to as the silent "killer fats." Next time you go grocery shopping, please take the time to check the ingredients of the food product for these ingredients. Trans fats should not be part of either your "old" diet plan at any time and certainly not part of your "new" diet plan.

b) Energy Drinks - The Legal Drug

As a fitness coach, I can almost regularly observe other athletes consuming their energy drinks before, during, or after workouts. You may be wondering why they should be avoided. Let me be very clear about that: These energy drinks represent nothing more than an addictive drug, filled to the brim with sugar, artificial flavors, and caffeine. To this day, caffeine is considered an underrated addictive substance. Of course, one or two cups of coffee a day will not harm anyone. However, these energy drinks contain "tons" of sugar and plenty of caffeine. The risk of becoming addicted to caffeine is therefore particularly high due to the regular intake of these drinks. Manufacturers of such energy drinks are particularly clever in their approach: As soon as they have reached the legally permissible limit for the admixture of caffeine, they add the so-called "guarana extract." Ultimately, this is also just caffeine, so the caffeine content increases again as a result. However, since this caffeine is derived from an extract and the blending process is different than that of caffeine, this additional caffeine blending in the form of this extract is considered perfectly legal. Strictly speaking, people who regularly consume these energy drinks are therefore actually drinking more caffeine in many cases than would be legally permissible.

Caffeine is an extremely stimulating stimulant. It can keep you awake and active for a long period. However, in high doses, it can cause high blood pressure, paranoia, heart attacks, and even panic attacks. If you should find a low-sugar energy drink with a moderate amount of caffeine and don't want to give it up, go for it. However, I recommend that you keep your hands off it altogether. After all, what's written on the package insert doesn't necessarily make up the contents.

c) Milk – The Underlying Cause of Many Health Issues

The diagram of the food pyramid at the beginning of chapter 5 unfortunately contains a disastrous dietary recommendation of the "Food and Drug Adminstration", which is the advocacy of moderate consumption of dairy products. Dairy products should be avoided completely if possible, because milk from animals is significantly different from breast milk. Humans are not designed to consume animal milk. Please do not be fooled by commercials that milk is healthy! It is not only a lie, but the exact opposite is the case. The dairy industry invests billions worldwide every year to keep up this pretense. But appearances are deceiving, and they are deceptive at your expense, and by that I mean primarily the health costs you are putting up with. The only milk that is truly healthy is *breast milk*. Animal milk contains three times as much protein as breast milk. This alone can cause metabolic disorders and affect the health of your bones. One of the dairy industry's most dangerous lies is that milk contains calcium, which is responsible for keeping bones healthy. Nothing could be further from the truth: When you drink animal milk, your body becomes "acidic," meaning your *pH value* changes. The pH measures the acid-base content of your body. An optimal pH should be around 7. However, the range can be anywhere from 1 to 14. To rebalance this excess acidity, calcium must be released from your bones. This, in turn, leads to a weakening of your bones, whose health depends significantly on this calcium. This can lead to a reduction in bone density and eventually osteoporosis. As you can see, consuming animal milk does not contribute to the health of your bones. In fact, it does just the opposite. Animal milk does contain calcium. However, this calcium is not calcium that the body can utilize. However, an **over-acidified** body triggers other adverse health effects, such as the following:

a) Acidosis makes nutrient absorption difficult or slows it down.

b) It suppresses the activity of the immune system.

c) It promotes listlessness.

d) It weakens the self-healing powers of the body.

e) It contributes to hormonal fluctuations and hormonal imbalances.

f) It contributes to premature aging.

g) It slows down the digestive process.

An **alkaline** body, on the other hand, has very beneficial effects on health:

a) It promotes the self-healing powers.

b) It strengthens the immune system, reducing susceptibility to disease.

c) It contributes to a young healthy skin appearance, promoting a more youthful appearance.

d) It enables deeper and more restful sleep.

e) It makes active and more energetic.

f) It reduces the risk of developing arthritis, osteoporosis and cancer.

g) It increases the ability to concentrate and mental strength.

h) It supports weight reduction

As you can see, pH plays an essential role in a whole range of processes in your body. Let's come back to animal milk or the factory farming that is often associated with it: Factory farming in agriculture is also known for literally "stuffing" the animals with antibiotics to prevent the animals from getting sick. The animals' diet consists of industrially processed and genetically modified grains. If you drink animal milk, you can expect these "nutritional ingredients" to become part of your diet. Dairy products have a devastating effect on your digestive system over time. This is because for the human body to digest and utilize *lactose* (milk sugar), it needs a certain enzyme to do so, namely *lactase*. However, this very important enzyme is <u>no </u>longer produced in the human body after the end of the 6th year of life at the latest. In some people, this is even the case after the end of the 3rd year of life. However, since most people continue to consume animal milk after this age, lactose can no longer be digested by the human body. It therefore remains undigested in the body and accumulates in the intestines. This often leads to cramps, bloating, nausea, diarrhea, tonsillitis, asthma, ear infections, allergies, acne, strep throat, skin irritations and weight gain. Dairy products also contain the protein *casein*. Studies have shown that this protein strongly promotes the growth of cancer cells. So, please stay away from dairy products.

5.2 What You Can Enjoy in Moderation!

Eating in moderation is a key element to a successful diet plan. There is a whole range of delicious foods. You don't have to give them up completely. People who want to lose weight sometimes fail at the very resolution because they believe that they are now expected to eat only raw vegetables and grains all day. Each of us enjoys a chocolate bar or a piece of cake every once in a while. That's why things that taste good to you are allowed to be part of a healthy lifestyle because these things often help reduce stress. The most important thing is that you enjoy in moderation! Eating a piece of chocolate cake on the weekend is absolutely fine. However, if you do that every day, your cholesterol levels will increase dramatically and so will your risk of a heart attack. On the other hand, your craving for these and similar foods may well start to decrease. This is because many people who have started to change to a low-fat diet start to get sick if they consume very fatty foods at the same time. Your body just can't handle an inconsistent change in diet very well.

a) Soft Drinks

Soft drinks (non-alcoholic beverages) are nowadays an integral and indispensable part of the fast-food society. Soft drinks are foods that are classified as food products that should be avoided altogether. Therefore, they should only be drunk in exceptional cases, because they belong to the unhealthy stimulants.

The problem with most soft drinks is that they are virtually "stuffed" with sugar. This causes them to extract even more water from the body. Soft drinks, therefore, don't really quench thirst but contribute to getting thirsty again quickly. As sugar is consumed in the form of liquid allows the sugar to be absorbed (assimilated) by the body very quickly. However, the body is not designed for such a rapid release of carbohydrates. The body responds to this "sugar invasion" by producing large amounts of insulin in the pancreas to utilize the sugar and thereby lower blood sugar levels again. However, this is only partially successful and the rest of it is converted into fat. You should also be aware that when soft drinks are consumed, the blood sugar level not only rises rapidly but also drops sharply again after the body has processed the sugar. The abrupt drop in blood sugar levels after some time can therefore also generate lethargic states in some cases. Incidentally, this connection also applies to white flour, potatoes, and white rice, since these products contain only the so-called *simple* carbohydrates. For this reason, you should also avoid these products if possible. Therefore, rather resort to sweet potatoes, wholemeal flour, and brown rice.

You should also be aware that sugar is the primary food source for cancer cells. Cancer cells cannot survive without sugar. The strong insulin production when sugar is ingested also promotes the growth of cancer cells. Even though soft drinks are certainly very delicious, they should therefore only be consumed in very small quantities for the reasons given above. Considering that there are alternatives that are just as delicious, but without negative health effects, it should not be too difficult to give them up. Flavored water is certainly one of them. It has no calories and there are several sorts of flavors. There should be something for every taste. Other suitable drinks are apple juice spritzers (1 part juice: 3 parts water), fruit juice spritzers, mineral-rich still mineral water, fruit and herbal teas, and tea lightly sweetened with honey (1 teaspoon per 100mL).

b) Fats, Oil, Protein, and Sugar

First of all, I want to make it clear that your body relies on fat to perform its bodily functions. However, this amount of fat that your body needs is far less than most consume. You can find valuable fats in nuts (almonds, cashews, walnuts, Brazil nuts) and seeds (sesame seeds, flax seeds, sunflower seeds, pumpkin seeds). Oil is also basically just fat. A lot of people try to make a distinction here, but ultimately oils are just another form of fat. They only differ in how they are used. Oils usually contain cholesterol. There are two different types of cholesterol: HDL and LDL. LDL is the "bad" cholesterol. It clogs the arteries, which can lead to very serious health issues, such as heart disease. HDL is the "good" cholesterol. It is not only necessary for the smooth functioning of the body but also lowers the "bad" cholesterol (LDL). You should therefore consume oils and fats containing LDL cholesterol only very rarely. Therefore, use much more often oils that contain HDL cholesterol, such as olive oil, sunflower oil, rapeseed oil, linseed oil, and walnut oil. However, please keep in mind that these oils are still fats, too. Although they help lower your "bad" cholesterol, they still remain fat and therefore lead to gain weight. My secret tip to all those who don't only want to keep their weight under control but also want to make a significant contribution to their health at the same time: *Coconut oil*. The health effects of coconut oil are unprecedented:

a) It does <u>not</u> contain cholesterol!

b) It stimulates the metabolism and thus contributes to weight loss.

c) The *lauric acid* contained in coconut oil strengthens the immune system and thus promotes resistance to diseases, including cancer.

d) It contributes to the maintenance of thyroid and bone health and promotes mineral absorption.

e) It has antifungal effects, thereby reducing the susceptibility to fungal attack.

f) Its antiviral, antibacterial, and antimicrobial properties have an anti-inflammatory effect.

Several studies have been conducted among the inhabitants of the Pacific Islands as coconut oil is an essential part of their diet. Those studies found out that those among them who cover 30%-60% of their calories through the intake of coconut oil, showed almost no traces of the cardiovascular disease. Incidentally, top models such as Victoria Secret and Miranda Kerr are huge advocates of coconut oil and even admit that coconut oil has played a crucial part in achieving and maintaining their dream figure. If you value the highest quality and purity when choosing coconut oil, I recommend "Extra Virgin Coconut Oil". However, make sure that it is an organic product.

Valuable animal proteins are found in sea fish (mackerel, herring, tuna, salmon), in eggs, and in lean meat (e.g. beef). Valuable vegetable proteins can be found in cereals (spelt, oats, bulgur) and in legumes (lentils, peas, beans, etc.).

Refined sugar, sweets, and desserts should only be consumed in rare exceptional cases. Regular consumption of refined sugar and fat leads to obesity, which also significantly promotes the development of diseases such as diabetes. Rather, to satisfy your appetite for sugar, turn to foods such as *brown sugar, natural honey,* or *maple syrup.* Make sure that no extra sugar has been added to these foods. That's because sugar can be found even in foods where you wouldn't expect to find it, such as salad dressings, sauces, cereals, breakfast cereals, and even spice mixes. But there are other awesome alternatives, such as *stevia, dates,* or *coconut blossom sugar.* Stevia is a plant that grows in South America. And although stevia is about 200 times sweeter than conventional sugar, it does not lead to excess insulin production in the pancreas with its negative consequences already mentioned. For diabetics, cancer patients, people suffering from yeast infections, or even people who want to keep their blood sugar levels under control, stevia is the perfect alternative. However, please make sure to buy organic products. These are wonderful alternatives to refined sugar, fats, and sweets. Even (sweet) fruits contain some sugar in the form of fructose. Therefore, you should also enjoy them in moderation. However, high-fiber fruits contain higher-quality carbohydrates that are much better utilized by the body and are therefore converted to fat to a much lesser extent. Choose fresh fruits that are not dried or preserved. The nutrient content of these fruits is much higher. If you buy canned fruit, make sure it has a natural content.

5.3 What Should Make Up the Bulk of Your Diet!

If you heed the advice from the last two chapters, you have already taken an important step in the right direction. However, you may be wondering what should make up the bulk of your diet instead if you are challenged to avoid some foods completely and eat others only in moderation. In this chapter, I would like to answer that question. However, the following list does not claim to be complete. One can easily write a book about what an optimal diet should look like. I will therefore keep this list rather short but quite informative.

The majority of your diet should consist of high-quality (complex) carbohydrates and high-fiber foods. More than 45% of your total diet should contain grains (but not wheat). This is followed by vegetables and protein, each of which should make up 15% of your diet. Fruits should be included in your diet at a level of at least 12-15%. Oils, fats, and sugars should only make up 1-3% of your total diet. wever, this does not apply to coconut oil which can be consumed at will and without limits. So much for a rough overview. Let's go a little deeper now.

5.3.1 Wholemeal Bread

Whole grain or multigrain bread is an excellent source of fiber and high-quality carbohydrates, which are released slowly in the body and are therefore not usually converted into fat. You should avoid white bread at all costs. This bread contains only nutrient-poor carbohydrates and very little fiber. The greater the proportion of fiber and whole grains, the better.

5.3.2 Vegetables

When buying vegetables (and fruits), please make sure that they are organic, as non-organic vegetables and fruits are highly contaminated with pesticides. The following vegetables should definitely be included in your diet plan as they are rich in vitamins, minerals, fiber and antioxidants: Leafy greens, avocado, asparagus, beet, cabbage, carrots (are fat-soluble, so always eat with a dash of oil), cauliflower, celery, cucumber, garlic, lettuce, mushrooms, radishes, spinach, tomatoes, and zucchini. In addition, I would like to briefly point out a highly underrated vegetable: Beans. Beans are an excellent source of fiber, carbohydrates, and minerals. These carbohydrates are also released slowly in the body. They are even better than whole wheat bread! Unfortunately, they rather seem to have a bad "reputation" because of their "side effects", such as bloating. However, you shouldn't let that blind you to their excellent health benefits.

5.3.3 Brown Rice and Wholemeal Pasta

Brown rice is much healthier than white rice. Preparing it may take more time but it is rich in fiber. Whole-grain pasta is also much healthier than conventional pasta, which is usually made from wheat. Whole wheat pasta has also a lot of fiber and nutrients.

5.3.4 Fruit

Fruits such as apples, oranges, bananas, strawberries, blueberries, cranberries, raspberries, tangerines, grapes, grapefruits, honeydew melons, watermelons, pomegranates, papayas, peaches, pineapples, citrus fruits, dried fruits, guava, jackfruit, mangoes, and dragon fruit should be part of your diet. Fruit is very healthy. Most of our vitamins come from fruit, which is also usually rich in fiber. As mentioned earlier, (sweet) fruits also contain sugar in the form of fructose. Therefore, you should also enjoy them in moderation. Even though high-fiber fruits contain higher-quality carbohydrates that are much better utilized by the body and are therefore converted into fat to a much lesser extent, overindulgence can also adversely affect weight reduction.

5.3.5 Poultry and Fish

In case you are neither vegetarian nor vegan, fish should be on your menu at least once a week. Fish is just a prime example. It contains very high-quality proteins, is very low in fat, and contains healthy unsaturated fatty acids such as omega-3. However, you should be very careful about the source of the fish, as fish often contains traces of mercury, which can wreak havoc on your health in the long run. Mercury cannot be naturally broken down by the body, meaning it can linger in the body for several years and decades while remaining unnoticed. Studies have shown that Alzheimer's patients often had mercury in their bodies. Therefore, please do not underestimate this danger! Therefore, be sure to use a reliable source of supply. Fish has been a cornerstone of the Japanese way of life for centuries. A population that has an average life expectancy of more than 80 years. It is believed that this is attributed to the regular consumption of fish.

Chapter 6: Movement and Fitness

6.1 Principles

First of all, I would like to congratulate you: If you have read this far and heeded the dietary recommendations given, you have already taken a very decisive step towards not only losing weight successfully but also towards leading a much healthier life in the first place. As for the following chapters, I wish to also motivate you to do sports activities. Once you realize that if you couple your change of diet with sporting activity, the effects will be many times greater. If a sporting activity has not been part of your everyday life, you do not have to despair. It is not a matter of demanding top athletic performance from you from now on. In order to support you on your journey to pursue a healthy lifestyle and your desired weight as fast as possible, I have come up with a fitness plan for you at the end of this book. Just think of it as a coaching plan that you would go for if we were to work together.

6.2 Things to Know About Endurance Sports

Before we take a closer look at two important types of endurance, you should know the following context: *Endurance* is generally understood as **fatigue resistance**.

These fatigue symptoms can occur in very different ways:

a) *physical* fatigue

b) *mental* fatigue

c) *sensory* fatigue (this refers to a temporary reduction in sensory perception).

d) *motor* fatigue (this causes the central nervous system to temporarily limit the sending of movement impulses).

e) *motivational* fatigue

As you can see, the effects of fatigue vary greatly, which is why it is necessary to maintain fatigue resistance over a long period. So, how can fatigue resistance be achieved? Well, the activity of your muscles depends on an adequate supply of *energy* and *oxygen*. This energy is provided in the form of *glucose* (sugar), *glycogen* (multiple sugars), and *adenosine triphosphate* (ATP). ATP is considered the most important energy supplier to ensure the proper functioning of bodily functions that require energy. An adequate supply of ATP also improves metabolism, contributes to well-being, reduces recovery time, and ensures faster wound healing. To put it bluntly: Without sufficient ATP, nothing in the body can function smoothly! However, the activity of the muscles is not only dependent on a sufficient supply of energy and oxygen because a sufficient supply of energy and oxygen requires the waste products (carbon dioxide, water, lactic acid) produced during metabolism to be also removed via the bloodstream of the cardiovascular system at the same time. Endurance sports have the following effects on the body:

a) Your vascular system becomes stronger, increasing nutrient and oxygen supply and decreasing your susceptibility to vascular disease.

b) The blood becomes thinner and the blood volume can increase by up to 25%, i.e. by 1-2 liters. This in turn causes an increase in red blood cells, which increases the transport capacity of oxygen.

c) Breathing works more efficiently, causing an increase in performance.

6.3 Are You In Shape? Let's Find Out!

Any fitness coach who wants to draw up an individual fitness plan for his students must first get an accurate picture of the student's current physical condition. Only then he can prepare a fitness plan perfectly tailored to the respective student. *Heart rate can be* used as a very reliable indicator to determine a student's cardiovascular fitness. Provided that there are no orthopedic restrictions, the so-called "knee flexion test" has proven to be a method that can be performed quickly and provides immediately reliable results. Proceed as follows:

1. Determine your **resting pulse**: Measure it immediately after waking up in the morning. However, you can also measure it after lying down for 10-15 minutes in a relaxed position. As for this method and the following pulse measurement, the pulse must be measured for one minute.

2. Measure your **stress pulse**: You will need to determine the stress pulse immediately after you have completed the exercise. The exercise consists of 30 squats in 60 seconds.

3. Measure your **recovery pulse**: You need to measure the recovery pulse one minute after the end of the exercise, i.e. 60 seconds after the end of the activity.

Then sum up the measured pulse beats!

5. Your stress index is then calculated as follows:

Sum minus 200 = stress index.

Use the following chart to evaluate your cardiovascular pulse capacity:

Pulse (stress index)	Rating
0-4	very good
5-8	good
9-12	moderate
13-15	weak
over 15	endangered

The pulse can be used to determine the heartbeats per minute. You should measure the pulse with the help of the index, middle, or ring finger (not with the thumb, as the thumb has its "own" pulse) on the carotid artery or wrist. To ensure the most accurate pulse measurement possible, it is best to proceed as follows:

Beats counted in 10 seconds times 6 = heartbeats per minute

<u>or</u>

Beats counted in 15 seconds times 4 = heartbeats per minute

<u>Important:</u> The maximum heart rate for men is 220 minus age. For women, it is 225 minus age. From the following heart rate table by age, you can get a pretty good idea of how heart rate activity affects your body.

AGE	BEGINNER 60% - 70%		INTERMEDIATE 70% - 80%		ADVANCED 80% - 90%	
	Beats/min	Beats/10 sec *	Beats/min	Beats/10 sec *	Beats/min	Beats/10 sec *
to 19	121 - 141	20 - 24	141 - 161	24 - 27	161 - 181	27 - 30
20 - 24	119 - 139	20 - 23	139 - 158	23 - 26	158 - 178	26 - 30
25 - 29	116 - 135	19 - 23	135 - 154	23 - 26	154 - 174	26 - 29
30 - 34	113 - 132	19 - 22	132 - 150	22 - 25	150 - 169	25 - 28
35 - 39	110 - 128	18 - 21	128 - 146	21 - 24	146 - 165	24 - 28
40 - 44	107 - 125	18 - 21	125 - 142	21 - 24	142 - 160	24 - 27
45 - 49	104 - 121	17 - 20	121 - 138	20 - 23	138 - 156	23 - 26
50 - 54	101 - 118	17 - 20	118 - 134	20 - 22	134 - 151	22 - 25
55 - 59	98 - 114	16 - 19	114 - 130	19 - 22	130 - 147	22 - 25
60 - 64	95 - 111	16 - 19	111 - 126	19 - 21	126 - 142	21 - 24
65 - 69	92 - 107	15 - 18	107 - 122	18 - 20	122 - 138	20 - 23
70 - 74	89 - 104	15 - 17	104 - 118	17 - 20	118 - 133	20 - 22
75 - 79	86 - 100	14 - 17	100 - 114	17 - 19	114 - 129	19 - 22
80 - 84	83 - 97	14 - 16	97 - 110	16 - 18	110 - 124	18 - 21
85 +	81 - 95	14 - 16	95 - 108	16 - 18	108 - 122	18 - 20

You need to read the table as follows: The term **"Beginner"** represents students who "only" aim at going for **fat burning** while doing endurance sports. So, if you should be between 30-34 years old and only want to go for fat burning, your heart rate needs to range between 113-132. In order to keep control over your heart rate during endurance sports, you need to have a heart rate monitor. Any sports watch uses to have a heart rate display.

The term **"Intermediate"** represents students who go for **aerobic exercises**. These exercises are more strenuous. Students who do these exercises don't go only for fat burning but strive to significantly improve their endurance. So, if you should be between 45-49 years old and want to do aerobic exercises in order to improve your endurance, your heart rate needs to range between 121-138. We will cover the character of these exercises in the following chapter.

The term **"Advanced"** represents students who go for **anaerobic exercises**. These are not exercises that cover endurance sports but rather strength endurance. So, if you should be between 50-54 years old and want to do anaerobic exercises in order to improve your strength endurance, your heart rate needs to range between 134-151. The character of these exercises will be covered in the chapter following the next chapter.

6.4 Aerobic Exercises

Endurance sports are basically divided into **aerobic** and **anaerobic** exercises. Let's focus on aerobic exercises first: If the body can maintain physical stress for a long time and continuously, we speak of *aerobic* endurance. In this case, energy is obtained by burning carbohydrates and fats through oxygen. The decisive factor for this combustion process is therefore an adequate supply of oxygen for the muscle cell, i.e. the cardiovascular system and respiration must ensure an adequate supply of oxygen. If this should be the case, physical stress can be endured for a long period of time. Aerobic sports are classified among the so-called "low-impact activities". These include sports such as aerobics, , bodyfit, fitness gymnastics, ski gymnastics, step aerobics, jogging, long walks, swimming, and power yoga. Simply put, you could say that any sport that makes someone short of breath, or at least breathing harder, is aerobic sports. Aerobic sports are great for breaking down fat. However, fat is a much better source of energy than carbohydrates and it takes more than twice as long to burn fat than carbohydrates. With this in mind, aerobic sports, which can be performed over a long period and which provide an adequate supply of oxygen, are ideal for burning fat and thus reducing weight.

6.5 Anaerobic Exercises

Anaerobic sports are the opposite of aerobic sports. Anaerobic exercises are characterized by short, but very intense physical stress. However, the significantly higher physical stress intensity compared to aerobic sports implies that the body does not have enough oxygen available for the exercise, i.e. the muscle cells are not sufficiently supplied with oxygen. This results in so-called *oxygen debt*. The energy required must therefore be obtained from the burning of *glucose* because the *creatine phosphate* (KP) and *adenosine triphosphate* (ATP) *stores* are completely depleted once an anaerobic exercise exceeds 7 seconds. This in turn leads to the formation of lactic acid (lactate). This hyperacidity causes the muscles to fatigue more quickly. To put it simply: Anaerobic exercises mainly access carbohydrate stores for energy production. Fats are hardly burned because the body is not provided with enough oxygen to get its energy from burning fat.

Anaerobic sports are classified among the so-called "high-impact sports". These include sports such as weight lifting, pull-ups, push-ups, squats, hurdling, and short sprints. Therefore, if you want to lose weight successfully, you should focus primarily on aerobic sports, because only these provide the muscles with enough oxygen to burn fats. However, anaerobic exercises should also be part of your training program, as these exercises are excellent for building muscle, which will also lower your fat percentage. For this reason, I have also included anaerobic exercises in the fitness plan in chapter 8.

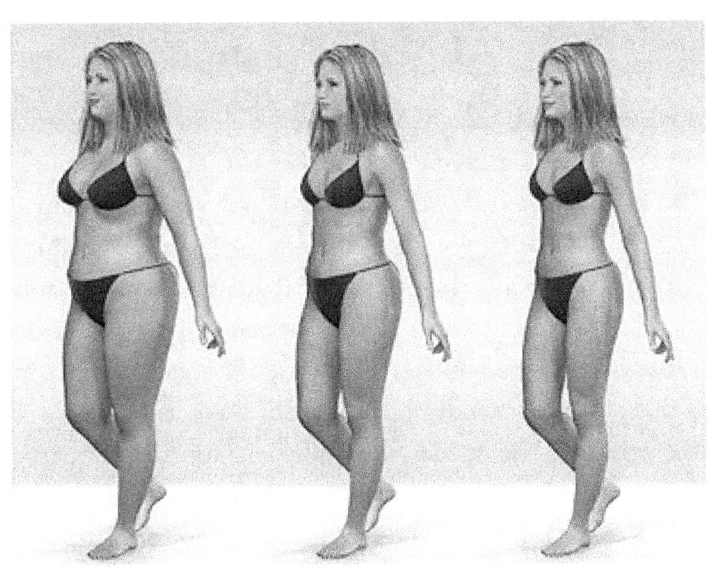

Chapter 7: How To Get Finally In Shape

7.1 Make a Plan

Regardless of what you want to achieve in life, the chances are significantly better if you have a plan. There's a saying that makes this connection pretty well: *"If you fail to plan, then you plan to fail."* Therefore, your goal of losing weight and finally getting fit is something you need to *plan for*. This is certainly not an easy undertaking, but it is probably the best proof that you are really serious about it. Most of us probably pursue either a full-time or at least part-time job, may also be married, and may also have a family. All of this, of course, requires our time and energy. With this in mind, therefore, you cannot leave it to chance to have some time for sports activities. You need to schedule your sports activities. Talk to your spouse or with your family about these sports activities, so that they also give you the necessary free space for it and you are not taken up for other matters during this time. If you can manage to schedule about 45 minutes of physical activity 2-3 days a week, that would be excellent and a very important step on your way to being permanently fit.

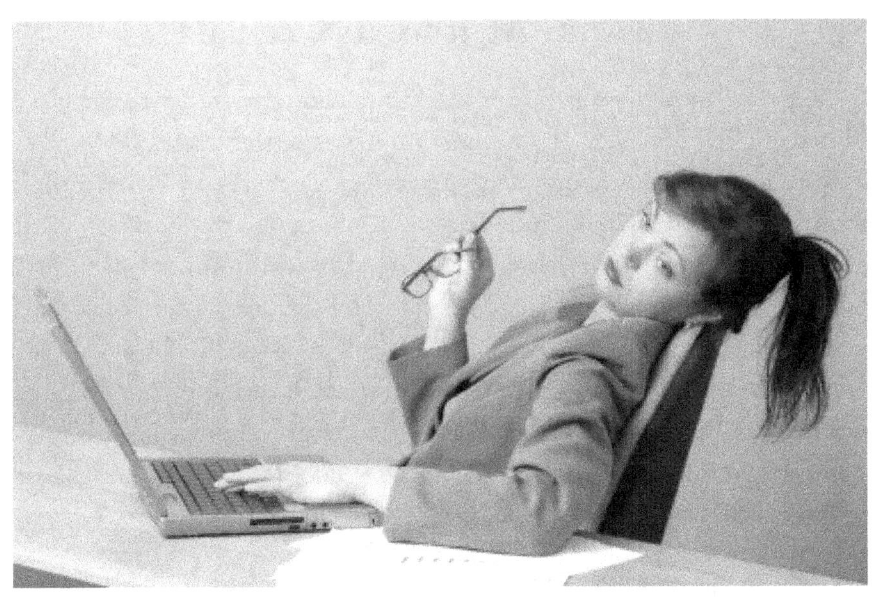

7.2 Your Attitude Is Crucial

First of all, the "good" news: If you work out regularly, you will achieve your goal of getting fit, regardless of whether you have the right attitude or not. This is simply the case because your body doesn't care whether you have the right attitude when you exercise or not. It only honors your physical commitment, but not your level of motivation. However, this commitment can diminish significantly over time if you lack the right motivation. Therefore, the right motivation can be the crucial key to long-term success. But how can you get motivated? For this purpose, I highly recommend **visualizing** your goals. As for me, I know of no better motivational boost than visualizing goals. This way even the powers of your subconsciousness are addressed and mobilized. The best way to do this is as follows:

a) Every day, imagine what you would like your ideal body to look like in the end. The picture at the beginning of Chapter 7 is not chosen at random. It is already an attempt to visualize your goal.

b) Imagine all the great activities you are going to do with your new body.

c) Imagine what it will feel like when you can buy clothes in your "desired" size.

d) Stick pictures of healthy foods and slim people you like to emulate on your refrigerator, wall, or anywhere else in your home. Design the background screen of your PC with such a photo. This way, you will stay motivated to keep pursuing your goal whenever you turn on the PC.

e) It is best to take about 5-10 minutes for this visualization before going to bed or after waking up.

Even though visualization is not a magic cure to lose weight or get fit, various scientific studies have shown that it improves the results and helps to increase motivation.

Tip of the day

Do not trust your scale

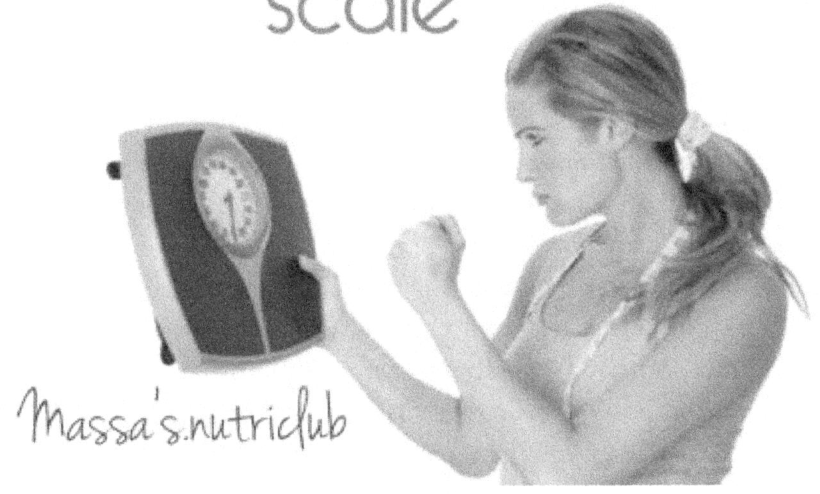

7.3 Do Not Be Discouraged By Occasional Setbacks

No one wants to suffer setbacks in life. However, if this should be the case though, please do not let them discourage you. Setbacks are part of life. Therefore, if you should fall back into your previous eating habits at short notice or "skip" your sports day, do not consider it a catastrophe. Just don't let this "slip" turn into a weekly, or even worse, monthly habit. So, check off this "slip" quickly and rather remind yourself of what you've already accomplished and not of this little "misstep." Also, look at setbacks as opportunities to learn from your mistakes. Learning from your successes is not nearly as effective as learning from your mistakes. For example, if you find that you can't make it through your workout on Friday evening as planned, pick a different day or time that day. So, learn from it, stick with it, and plan again.

If you manage to find a workout partner, it's not only another wonderful motivational channel but also another good way to better deal with setbacks. With him or her, you can share your triumphs but also your setbacks. Since he or she is on the same path, you can assume that he or she will support you to continue on your way. For the same reason, I also recommend that you join a Facebook group that deals with topics such as "Losing Weight Successfully", "Being Slim", "Workout" etc. These group members have the same goal as you. Their discussion posts contain the "ups" and "downs" along the way. These posts can and will encourage you to keep going and not give up because they will make you feel that you are not alone on your path. So, please do not underestimate the psychological value of a dynamic group community that shares the same goal as you. Most certainly, they will also appreciate your contributions to the discussion. As for my personal experience, I can assure you that I probably would have not achieved some goals that I had set for myself if it had not been for such a group. Therefore, don't let this opportunity go to waste!

7.4 All beginnings Are easy: Go For a Walk

If you have been avoiding sports activities for whatever reason, I recommend you start with walking. The best way to do this is as follows:

a) Choose a pleasant and safe walk.

b) Start walking at a slow pace.

c) Then after about 5 minutes, increase the pace to a "brisk" walk.

d) The intensity of your walk (easy, moderate, high) can be measured well by your heart rate. Therefore, you should measure it regularly during your walk. **Pulse watches** are excellent for this purpose. So, make sure to wear a pulse watch while walking and doing sports. In case you prefer to measure your pulse yourself, please remember the following rule of thumb:

Beats counted in 10 seconds times 6 = heartbeats per minute

<u>or</u>

Beats counted in 15 seconds times 4 = heartbeats per minute.

Whether the sporting activity, or as in this case, walking, represents a light, moderate, or high physical intensity depends on both the gender and the age of the person in question. Use the following <u>formula</u> as a basis for this:

<u>Maximum pulse (220 for men, 225 for women):</u>

1) Minus age times 0.65 = heart rate for **light** intensity

2) Minus age times 0.75 = heart rate for **moderate** intensity

3) Minus age times 0.85 = heart rate for **high** intensity

<u>Example</u>: A 27-year-old woman would like to go for a moderate sports activity. In this case, her heart rate should not exceed the following value:

225 (maximum pulse) - 27 (age) times 0.75 = 148.5

e) Take a 20-minute walk at a moderate to brisk pace about 3-5 times during the first week.

f) In the next week, increase the duration of the walk by 3-5 minutes. Proceed this way in each new week until the duration of your walk is 45-60 minutes in the end. Your goal should be to walk 5x per week.

g) Make sure you keep an upright posture when walking. Look forwards and not downwards. Pull your shoulders back and make sure they are relaxed while running.

h) While running, keep your elbows at a 90-degree angle to your body.

i) Make sure your shoes fit and are comfortable.

j) With moderate to high intensity walking measured by the formula given above, you will burn about 300 calories in 20 minutes.

After you have improved your endurance by walking, you can gradually move on to jogging. However, even then, please stick to these rules.

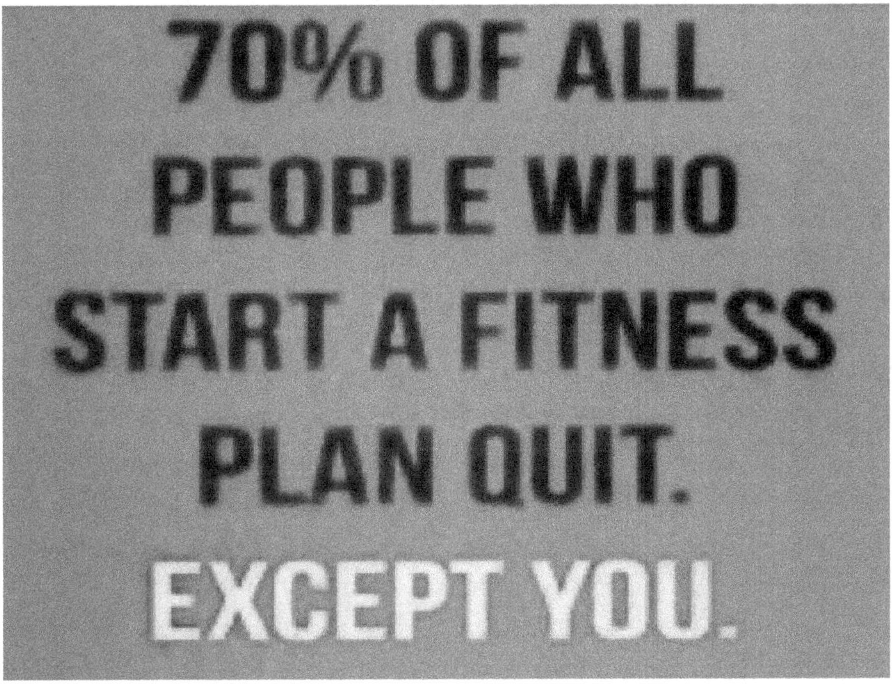

70% OF ALL
PEOPLE WHO
START A FITNESS
PLAN QUIT.
EXCEPT YOU.

Chapter 8: How Your Fitness Plan Could Look Like

8.1 The Warm-Up Phase

Every sports activity should start with a warm-up phase. Unfortunately, some people seem to underestimate this phase and use to skip it therefore - mostly for reasons of convenience. Why is this phase so crucial? Both your body and your psyche are not "water boilers" where you simply need to flip a switch to make the water boil in 60 seconds. Your organism and your psyche cannot adjust to a high physical intensity from one moment to the next. The warm-up phase, therefore, aims at generating the best possible physical and mental condition to slowly adjust you to the physical intensity ahead. However, this phase must not become a high-performance phase, i.e. you should not use more than 50% of your maximum power for the warm-up. Your maximum power is measured by your maximum heart rate (remember 220 for men and 225 for women) because warming up causes the oxygen demand in the muscles to increase, which, in turn, increases your breathing and heart rate. You might notice that this causes your breaths to become deeper and your blood pressure to rise. Oxygen intake can increase five to six times to about 8 liters per minute. Cardiac activity increases fivefold, so the heart pumps about 5.5 liters of blood per minute to the skeletal muscles. This strong blood supply to the muscles opens up their capillaries. In addition, significantly more synovial fluid is produced, making your joints suppler and more adaptable to the physical intensity ahead. At rest, the muscle temperature is about 89-93 °F. After the warm-up phase, it rises to 101 °F. By the way, I would also like to point out that you cannot increase the body temperature through a so-called "passive warm-up", such as showering or visiting the sauna. Unfortunately, this misconception still seems to exist.

Given the processes released in the organism during the warm-up, this phase should never be underestimated as it is a fundamental part of any training. Warming up helps to significantly reduce the risk of injury and increases both performance readiness and performance potential.

For example, activities such as brisk walking, running (jogging), cycling, or even movements to music are suitable for warming up.

8.2 The Workout Plan

The following workout plan is not just theory, but a workout plan that I have worked out for my *Bodystyling* courses. Some fitness centers also use to name this course *Bodyfit*, *Power Gymnastics*, *Ski Gymnastics,* or *Fitness Gymnastics.* However, these courses mentioned use to cover more or less the same exercises. These courses are usually classified as *Functional Gymnastics.* Every time I use to make up a workout plan, I make sure that I incorporate exercises that cover any part of the body. This way, participants can perform a total body workout (total body conditioning). With this in mind, I would like to cover these exercises in the following chapters. This plan has proven itself in its implementation. Therefore, I assume that you will also benefit from it.

8.2.1 Abdominal Exercises

If you want to lose weight successfully and also look fit at the same time, you need to do regular exercises to strengthen your abdominal muscles.

Let's start with an exercise designed to strengthen the **straight** abdominal muscles. This exercise is also known as a *crunch*. To do this, first lie flat on your back, place your legs with your feet at hip-width. Place your hands behind your head. However, do not pull on the head. There should still be a fist-wide space between the chin and the sternum, i.e. do not pull the head towards the sternum. Lift your upper body slightly off the floor and move your head toward your knees or straightened legs. You should be facing the wall as you go up. The elbows point outward and remain there throughout the movement, i.e., do not pull the elbows forward as you go up. The head should not move, i.e. do not bob your head back and forth when going up or down. Above all, please avoid jerky movements. Perform the movement slowly and in a controlled manner. Pay attention to small movements when going up. When you go up, your lumbar spine should not leave the ground, i.e. it always keeps contact with the ground. Pay attention to your breathing, i.e. exhale during the wearing part of the exercise and inhale during the relieving part of the exercise. So, doing this exercise, you need to exhale as you go up and inhale as you go down.

I recommend doing this exercise at the beginning with a so-called *fitness ball*. This should look like this:

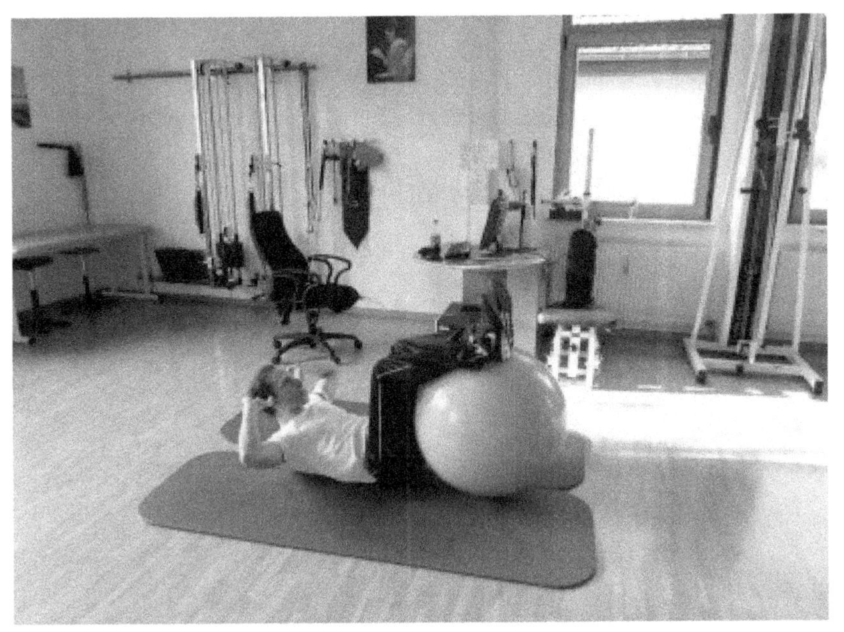

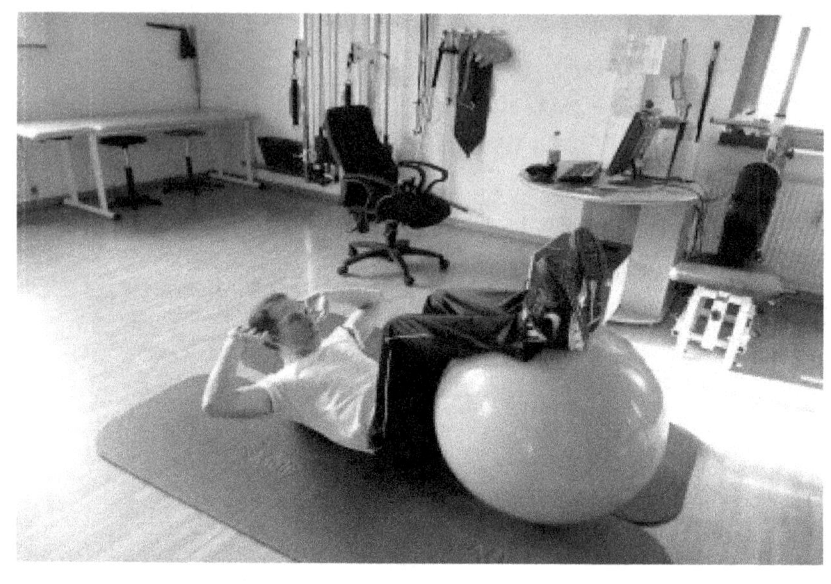

Unfortunately, strengthening the **lateral** abdominal muscles are often overlooked. The following exercise is very suitable for this: Lie on your side, bend your knees and hold your hands behind your head (again, do not pull on your head). Then, move your upper body towards your knees. The hands remain behind the head. Only the upper body moves forward in small (not jerky) movements. Make sure to follow the same rules as in the previous exercise: There should be a fist-width distance between the head and the sternum, i.e. do not rock the head back and forth and do not pull in the direction of the sternum. Most importantly, keep breathing while doing the exercise, i.e. exhale when going up and inhale when going down. Then switch sides after about 10 repetitions. The exercise should look like this:

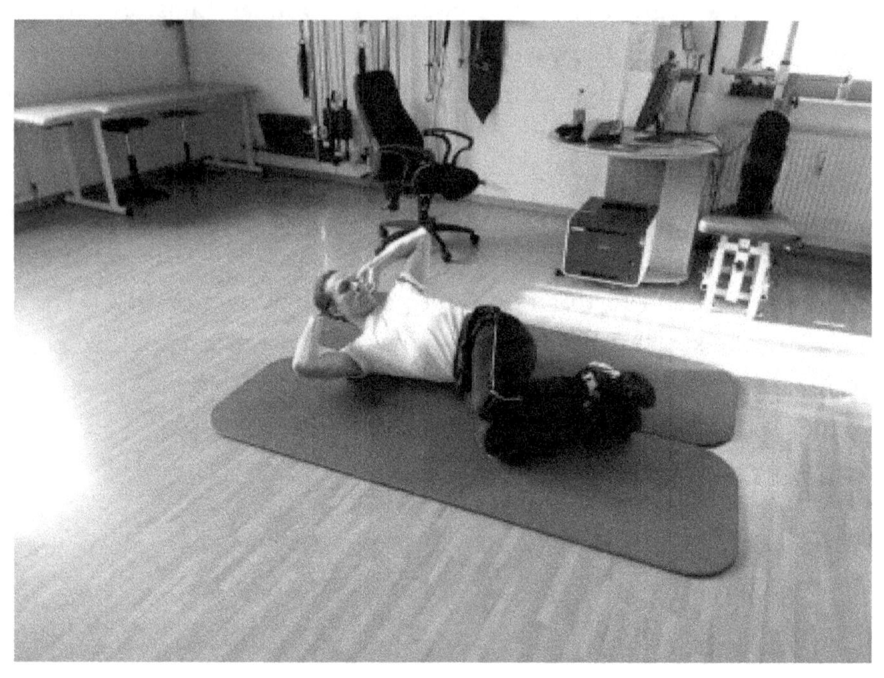

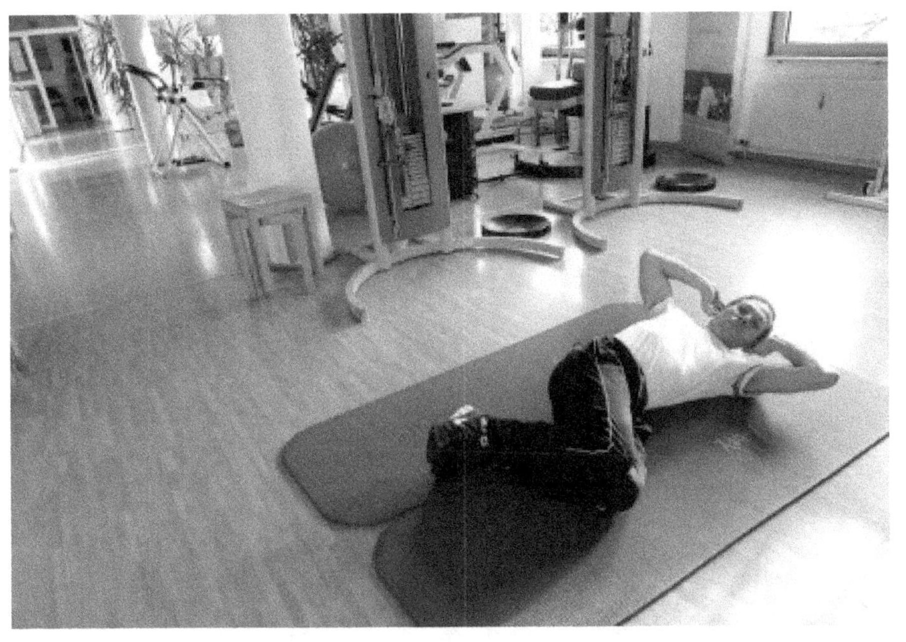

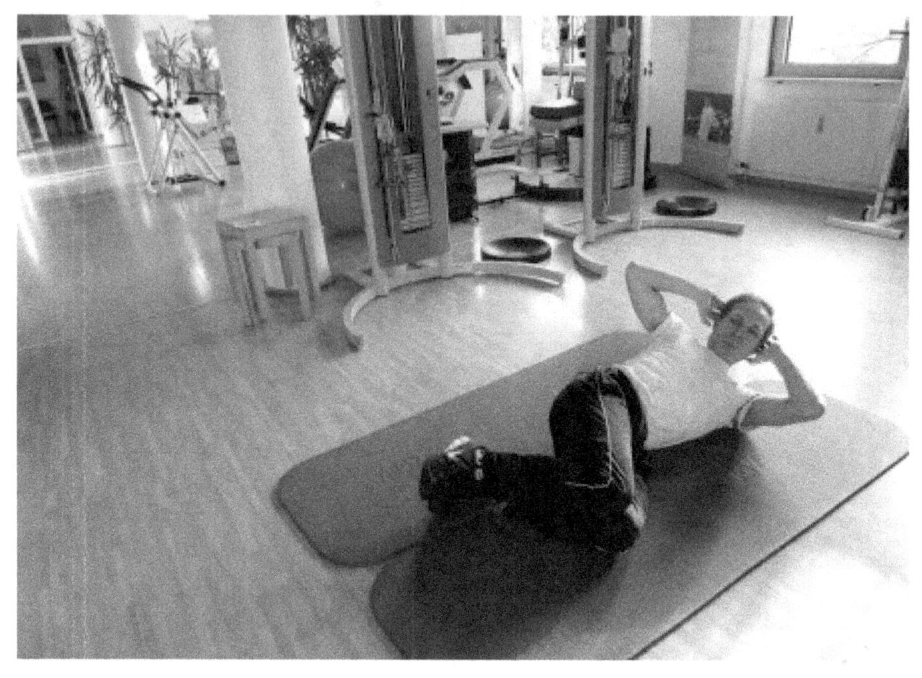

8.2.2 Exercise For Strengthening the Back

Your back health plays a crucial part in health, fitness, and resilience. The abdominal exercises from the last chapter contribute dramatically to strengthening your back. Simply put, you will never have a healthy back if your abdominal muscles are "flabby". Therefore, special courses focus primarily on back exercises. In order to strengthen your back, do the following exercise: First, get into the quadruped position. The knees should be under the hips and the hands under the shoulders. Then, stretch the right arm and the left knee *diagonally*, i.e. arm and leg are stretched crosswise. Then bring the right arm and left leg together under the body and then stretch them again. Make sure that the hips remain straight and the thumb points upwards. Tighten your abdomen as well, and most importantly, don't forget to breathe! Then, do the same exercise with your left arm and right leg. The exercise should look like this:

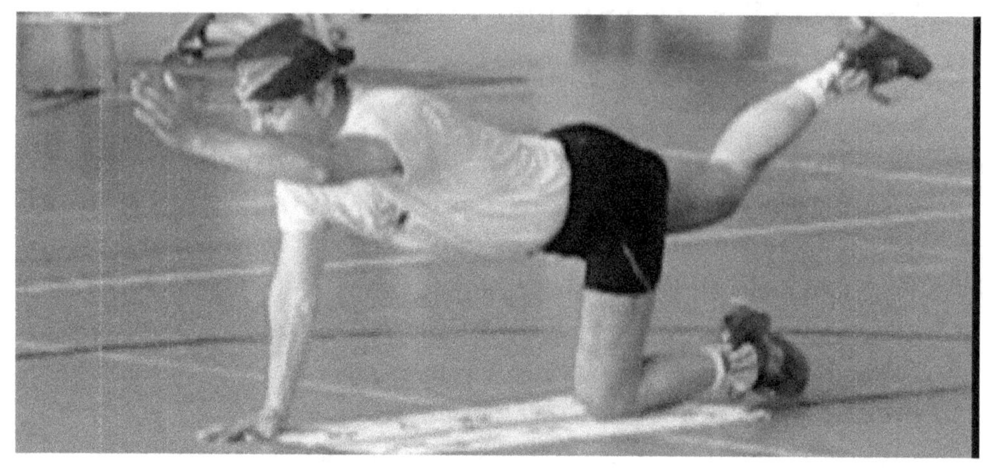

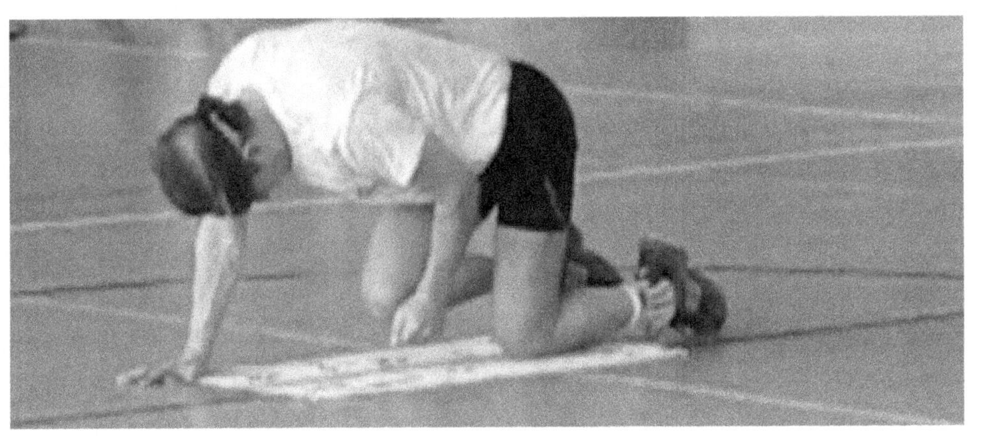

8.2.3 Exercise For Strengthening The Lateral Trunk Muscles

Strengthening the lateral trunk muscles should be a mandatory part of every training session. The best way to do this is as follows: Lie on your side and rest your forearm on the floor at a 90-degree angle with your elbow under your shoulder. Then, stretch out both legs and place them on top of each other with the tips of the feet pointing forward. Then, raise your hips until your torso lines up with your legs. The hips point forward. Hold the tension briefly before lowering the hips again. This exercise tenses the entire body. To increase this tension, you can also lift the upper leg and extend the hand towards the ceiling. Do 5-10 repetitions if possible. Then repeat the exercise with the other leg. The exercise should look like this:

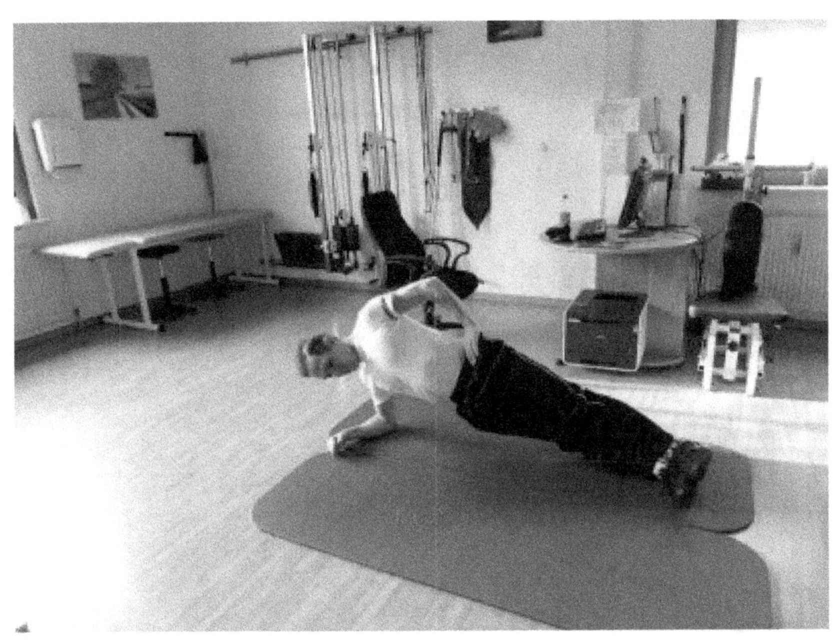

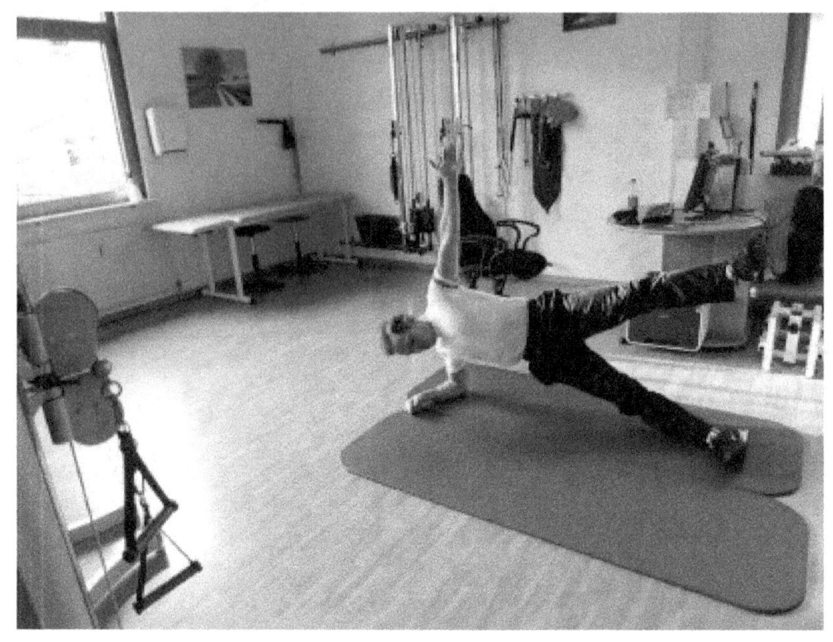

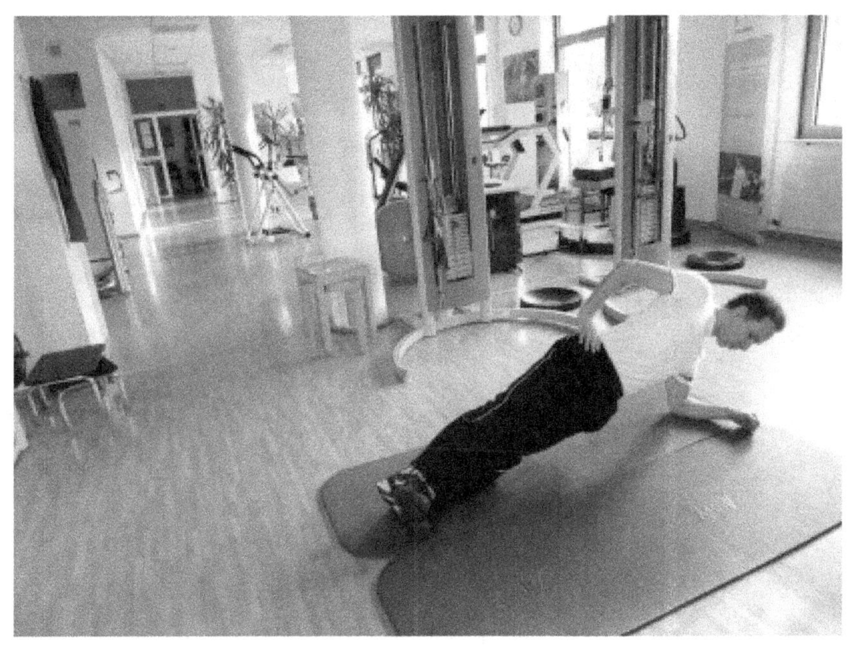

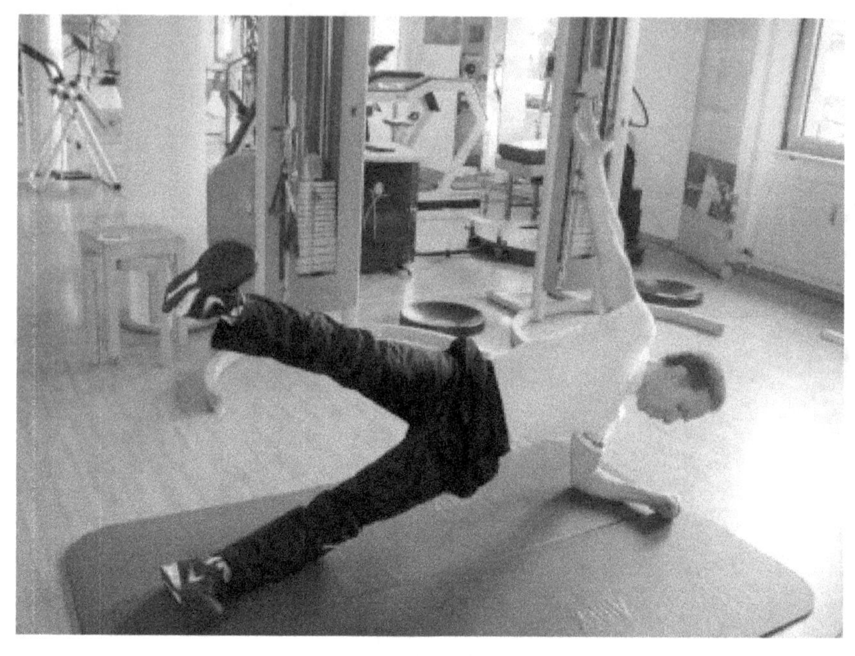

8.2.4 Exercise For Stretching The Lumbar Spine

Many people use to complain about pain in the area of the lumbar spine. That's why it is very important to do exercises for the lumbar spine regularly. For this purpose, I recommend the following excellent exercise: Lie flat on your stomach. Then bend your right arm at a 90-degree angle, with your head facing the direction of the arm that is bent at 90 degrees. Now pull the right leg diagonally to the left side of the body. Next, repeat the exercise with the left arm and leg. This is what the exercise should look like:

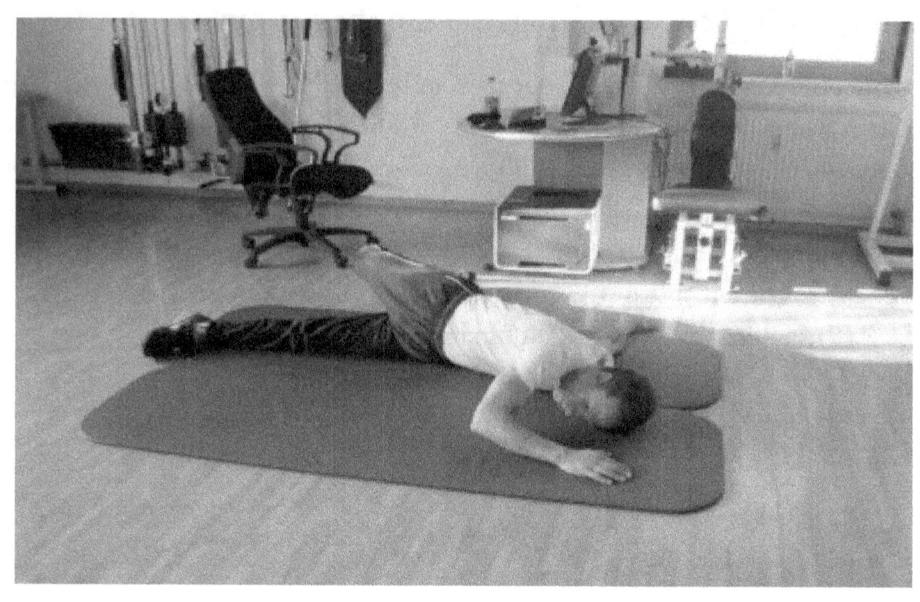

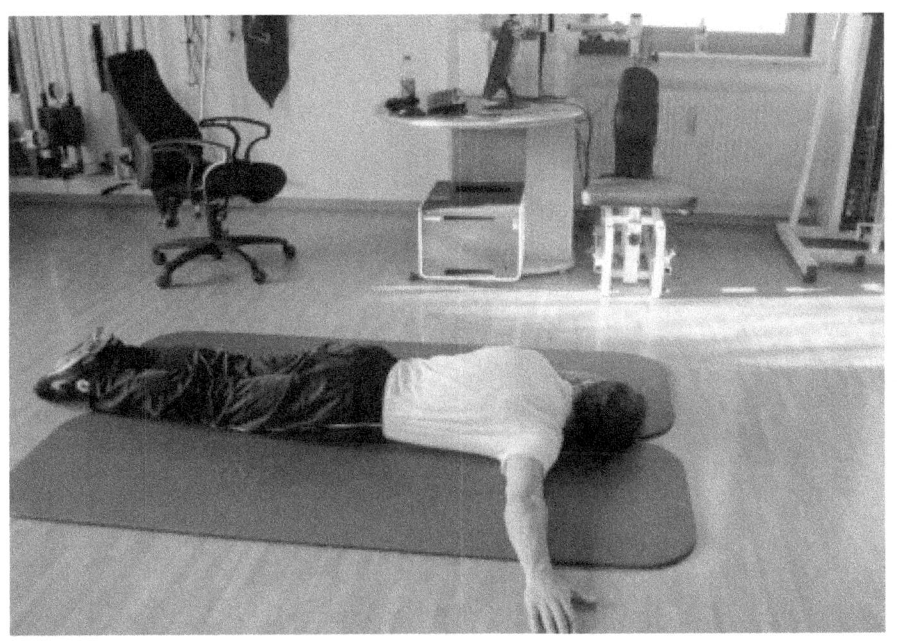

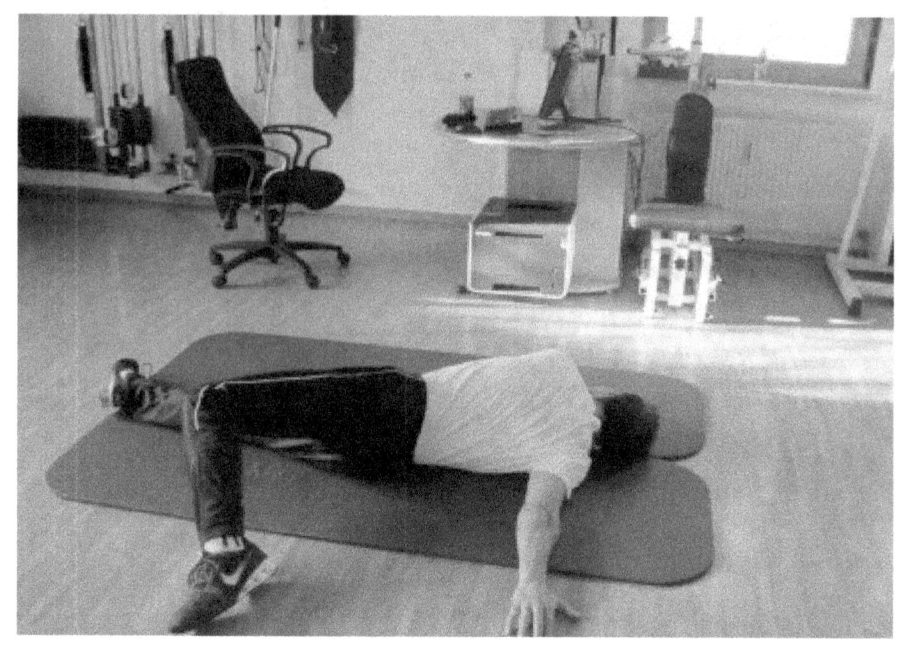

8.2.5 Exercise For Strengthening The Chest Muscles and Biceps (Forearm Flexors)

One of the best exercises to strengthen the chest muscles is push-ups. Proceed as follows: First, get into the quadruped position. Then, stretch your legs. Hold your hands under your shoulders at shoulder-width. Look down. Then, bend your arms as they go down with your upper body. Make sure that the upper body forms a straight line and that the head is in an extension of the spine, i.e. do not let the head hang or move it back and forth. Most importantly, keep breathing: When you go down, breathe in, and when you go up, breathe out. Also, make sure that you constantly tighten your abdomen while performing the exercise. If you find it too difficult to perform this exercise with your legs extended, then lower your knees and do the exercise with your knees lowered on the floor. This is what your posture should look like when doing push-ups:

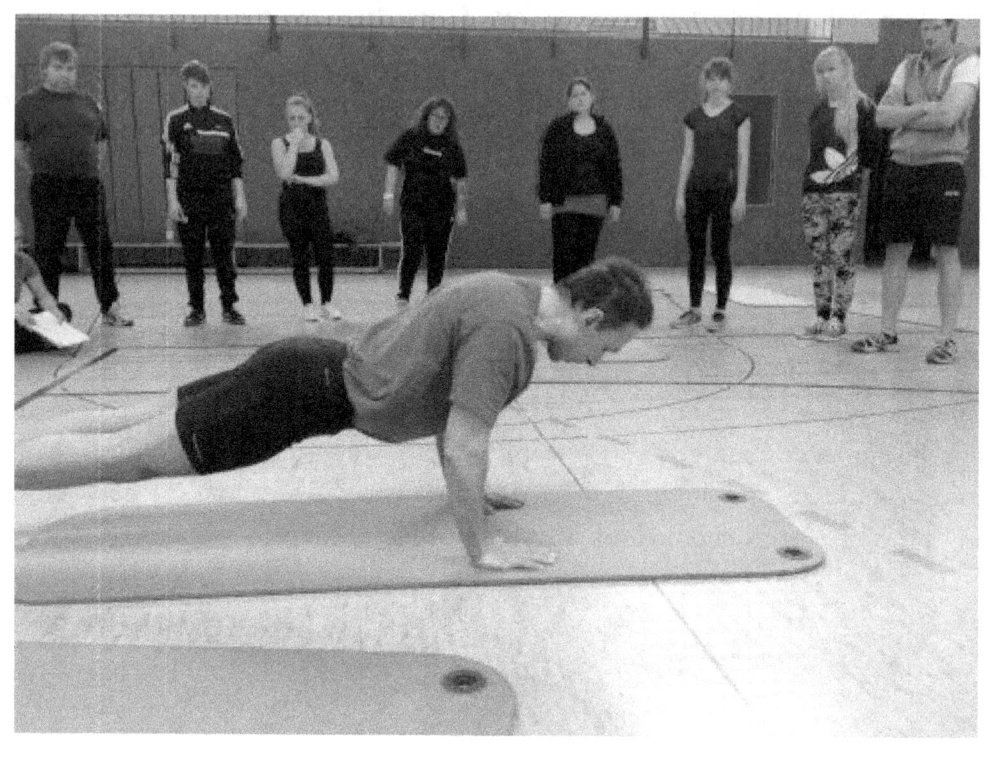

8.2.6 Exercise For Strengthening The Triceps (Forearm Extensors)

The muscles of the arms also include the so-called forearm extensors (triceps). These should also be strengthened regularly. To do this, you can adopt the position of the push-ups, changing only the position of the hands: Your hands should now <u>not</u> lie under the shoulders, but approximately *between the* hips and shoulders and point forward. This way, you train the triceps by going up and down. This is what the exercise should look like:

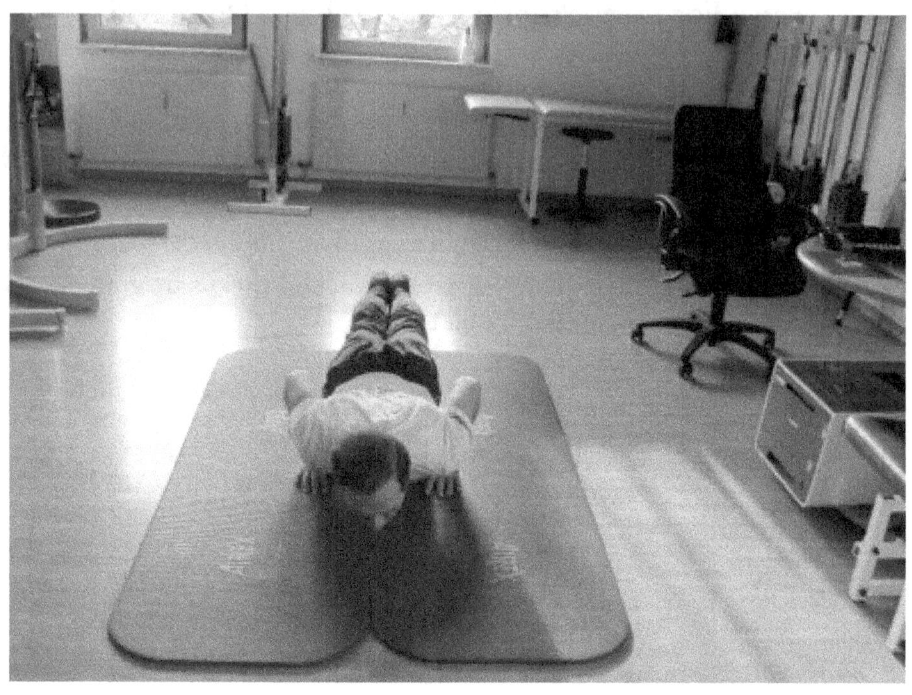

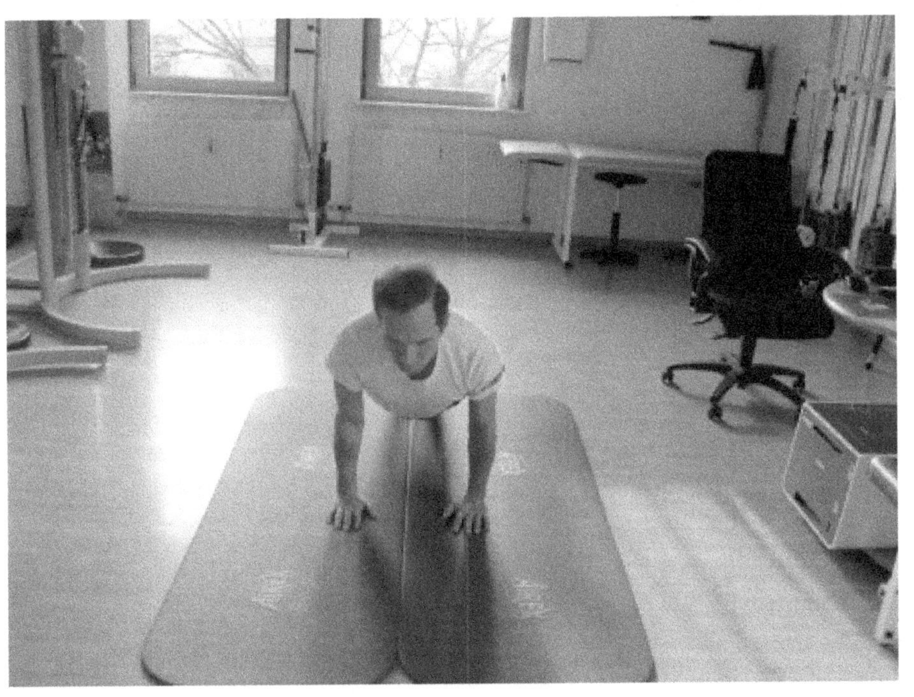

8.2.7 Exercise For Strengthening The Deltoids (Posterior Shoulder Muscles)

The push-up position is also great to strengthen these muscles. The only difference from the "classic" push-up position is that the hands point in*ward* instead of forward. This small variation alone shifts the emphasis of the exercise to the deltoids. This is what the exercise should look like:

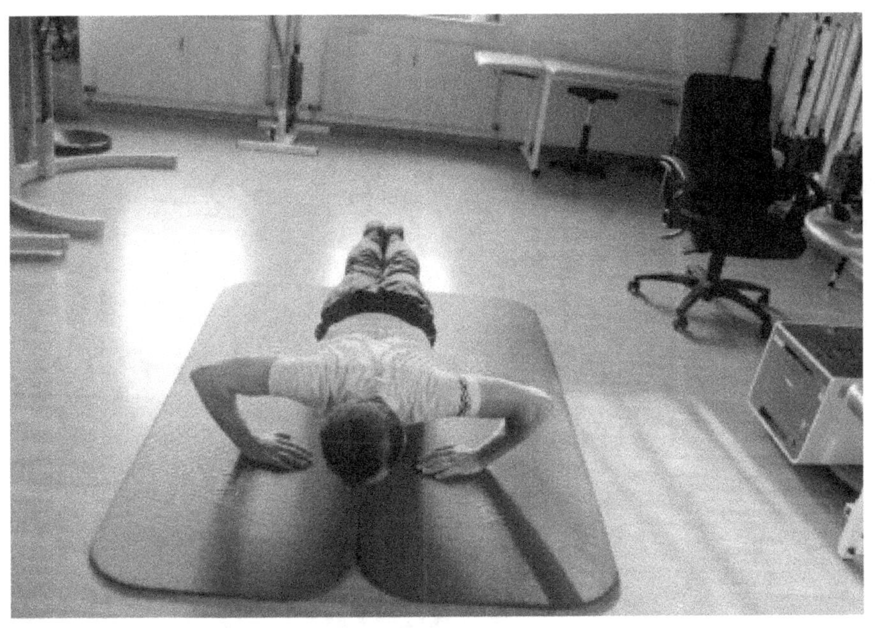

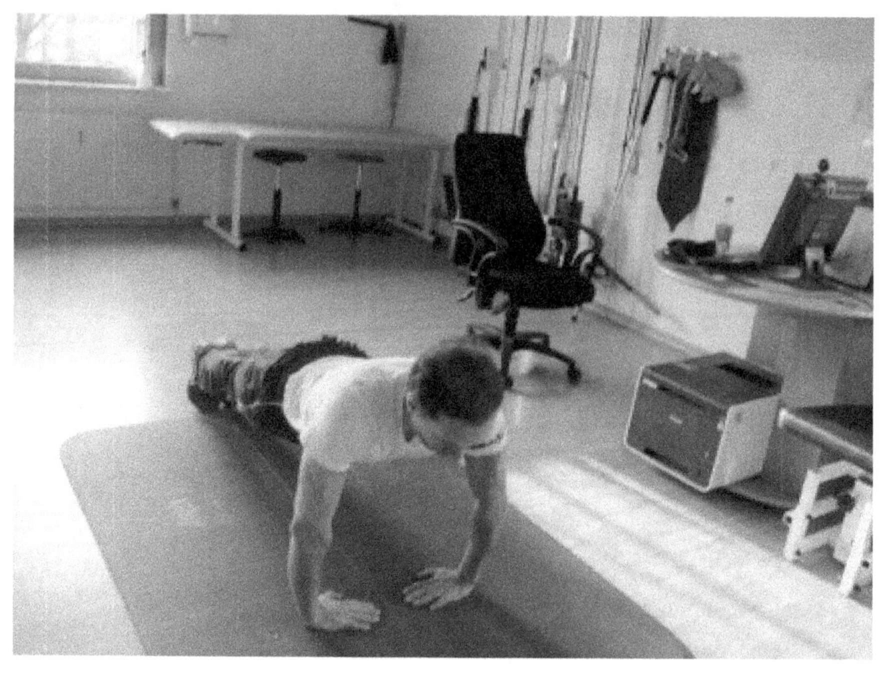

8.2.8 Exercise For Strengthening The Gluteal Muscles (Gluteus)

Weak and shortened gluteal muscles lead to a limited extension of the hip and thigh muscles. As a result, too much stress is being exerted on the knees. To avoid this, do the following exercise to strengthen the gluteal muscles: Lie flat on your back and stretch out your legs. Then, put both legs upright. Place the left leg on the right knee. Then, grasp the right knee with both hands. Then, slowly pull the right leg towards you in the direction of the chest. During this exercise, you will feel a stretch in the right buttock. Then, do the same exercise with your left knee. This is what the exercise should look like:

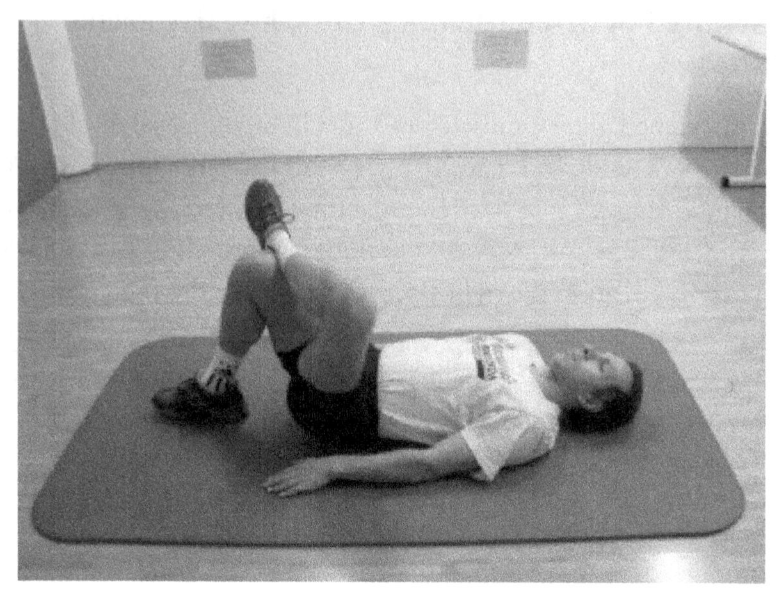

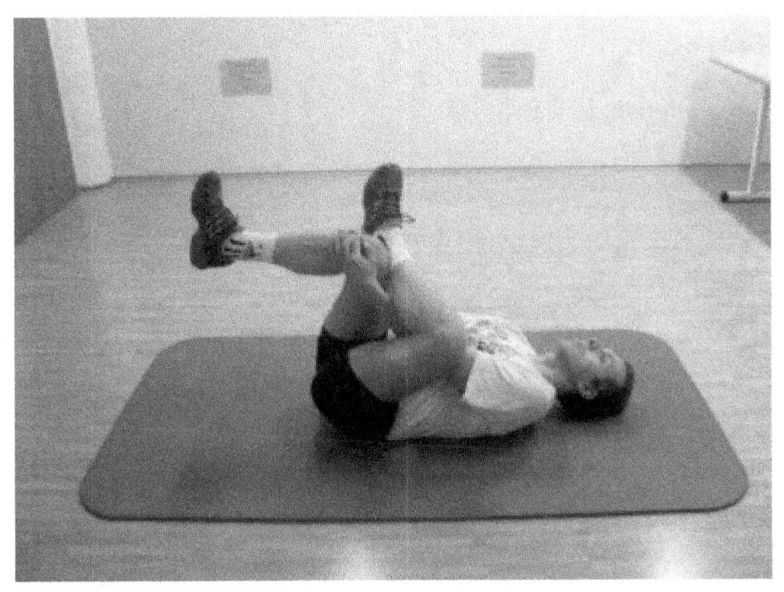

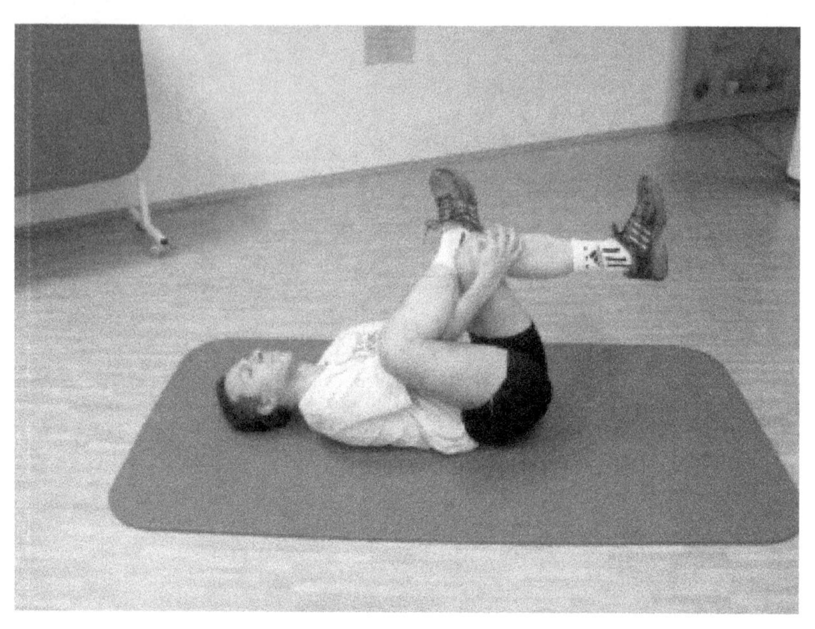

8.2.9 Exercise For Strengthening The Muscles of The Thighs and Hip Flexors

As mentioned in the last chapter, shortened gluteal muscles lead to a limited extension of the hip and thigh muscles. Therefore, the hip and thigh muscles should be strengthened by strengthening the gluteal muscles. Moreover, you can additionally strengthen the hip and thigh muscles by doing the following exercise:

First, stand upright. Then, bend your right leg and pull it toward your chest with both hands. Now grasp your right foot with both hands and pull your bent right knee behind your buttocks. Pull your abdomen in as you do so. Then, push your pelvis forward until you feel a stretch in your right thigh muscles. If you find it difficult to maintain your balance during this exercise, lean against the wall with one hand while pulling your right knee behind your buttocks with the other. Repeat this exercise with your left leg as well. This is what the exercise should look like:

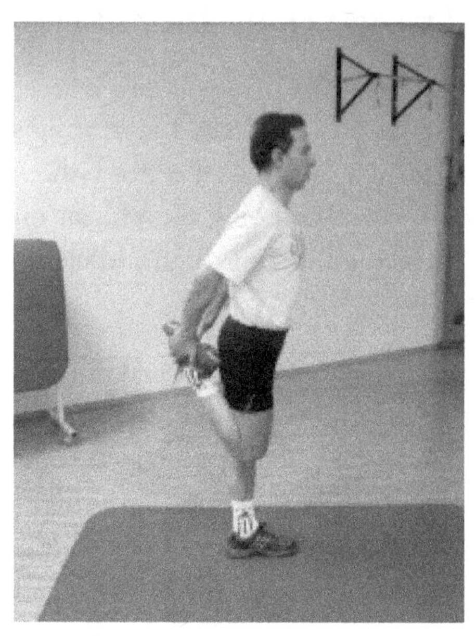

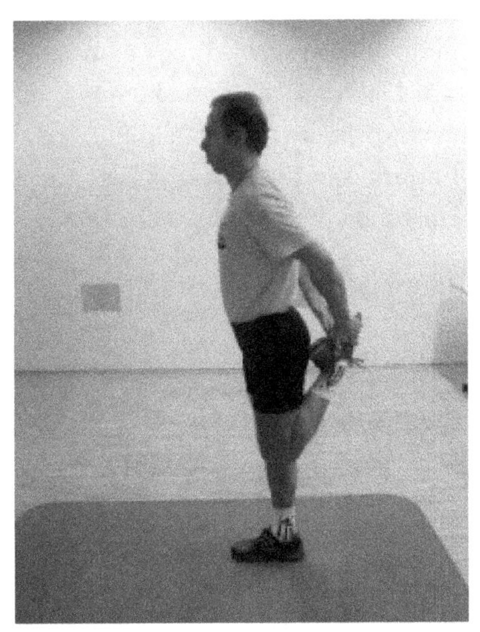

So, this is what your fitness plan could look like. If you can implement this plan, including walking, jogging, or cycling, into your daily routine twice a week, that would be a fantastic start. However, please make sure that you have at least one day break in between two workouts. This is because your body has regenerated about 90% after 12-18 hours. After 48 hours it has recovered to 100% again. I would like to give you the following *training principles:*

1. always increase the **training frequency** first!

2. then increase the **training scope!**

3. at last increase the **training intensity!**

Chapter 9: Final Thoughts

You might feel a bit overwhelmed after being "flooded" with an abundance of hints and tips. If this should be the case, this is okay. If I were your fitness coach and was allowed to look over your shoulder regularly to measure your progress, I would be able to better dose the flood of information presented in this book. I would first support you in changing your diet, as it has been described in the first chapters of this book. Then, I would make sure that you don't fall into the sneaky diet traps. After this, I would get you prepared to pursue a step-by-step workout plan specially tailored for you. However, unfortunately, since I cannot "take you by the hand" this way, my sincere wish associated with this book is to still guide you slowly but surely to your goal. You have set yourself an excellent goal, namely to stay healthy and get fit pursuing this diet and workout planner. Please don't let anyone discourage or dissuade you from finishing this "project". Surround yourself with people who will support you along the way. As for the fitness plan described in chapter 8, the number of repetitions for each exercise was deliberately set to a minimum. In the beginning, you set the pace (training frequency), then increase the training scope, and at last the training intensity. So, start slowly and increase gradually. Based on your measured heart rate (remember the table in chapter 6.3), you can very well measure the physical intensity of the individual exercises. So, based on your age you have learned about the heart rate you need to pursue for fat burning, aerobic, and anaerobic sports activities. You have also learned about the maximum pulse, which you must never exceed while working out.

Congrats! Note from the Author:

You've reached the end of the book!

Thank you for finishing **DIET AND WORKOUT PLANNER!**

Looks like you enjoyed it!

If so, would you mind taking 30 seconds to leave a quick review?

It would mean the **WORLD** to me!

I work hard to bring you books that you enjoy!

Plus, it helps and encourages me dramatically to produce more books like this in the future!

Also by Dr. Robertino Bedenian

Fitness Over 60 For Women – How to Stay Fit And Healthy As You Age

Does Back Pain Go Away? 10 Answers To The Most Acute Back Pain Issues

Massage Bible - A Beginners Guide To Western And Eastern Massage Therapy

Going Vegan - How To Vegan Without Going Crazy

Chiropraktik - Was Steckt Eigentlich Dahinter?

Massagen: Ein Überblick Über Westliche Und Östliche Massagetechniken

Natuerlich Abnehmen, Schlank Und Endlich Fit Sein

P.S. Ich Liebe Dich: Wenn Liebe So Einfach Wäre

Was Tun Bei Rückenschmerzen, Bandscheibenvorfall Und Ischiasschmerzen: 10 Antworten Zu Den Häufigsten Fragen Bei Rückenschmerzen

Was Tun Gegen Schlafapnoe, Schlafstörungen Und Schnarchen

Self-Help Books for Women – How to Overcome Depression, Anxiety, Divorce, Addiction, and Trauma

Your Super Gut Feeling Restored – How to Restore Your Life Energy and Overall Health from The Inside Out

Diabetes How to Help: Everything You Need to Know About Diabetes Type 1 and Type 2

Diet and Workout Planner: How to Stay Healthy and Get Fit for Life

Everything I Know About Love

The Sleep Easy Solution Book: How to Stop Sleep Apnea, Snoring, and Sleep Disorders

Watch for more at https://booksummarypublishing.com.

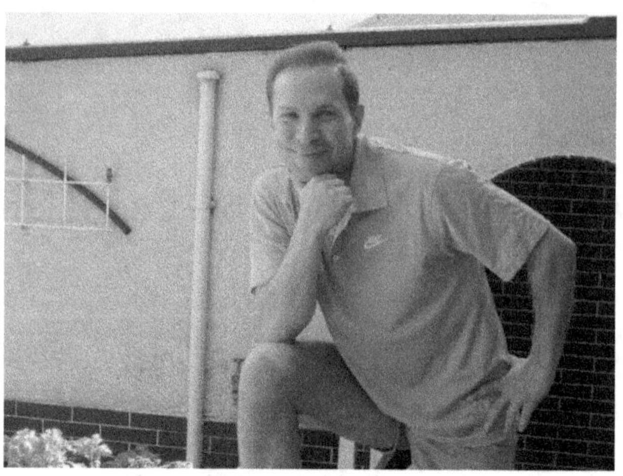

About the Author

Dr. Robertino Bedenian is a qualified fitness instructor accredited by the German Olympic Committee, a health and nutrition expert, and the author of several books on diet, health, and fitness!

For more than twenty years he has been a fitness coach at the sports university teaching aerobics, back gymnastics, stretching, high-intensity interval training (HIIT), power gymnastics, and athletic sports.

On his website, he has published more than 300 articles about the vegan lifestyle covering diet and health recommendations, detoxication programs,

fitness guidelines, and disease-related topics. He is part of a family with an orthopedic surgeon, a physical therapist, an osteopath, and an alternative practitioner.

He is also the founder of the brand "**Going Vegan**" selling high-quality supplements for optimal health.

You are more than welcome to check his website for more details: https://goingveganhealthbenefits.com.

His brand has been awarded continuously with 5-star feedback by customers for its outstanding product quality.

Dr. Bedenian is also the founder of the book company "**Book Summary Publishing**" publishing summaries and workbooks of Amazon #1 bestselling non-fiction books.

If you want to learn more about the summaries and workbooks that he has published so far, please visit his website: